'This book covers all the areas that I consider essential to my own and my patients' wellbeing – stress management, nutrition, work/life balance, present moment awareness, emotional wellbeing, physical health and efficient breathing. Providing evidence-based explanations and with useful practical exercises across all of these areas and more, it is essential reading for anyone who knows that there are elements of modern life that are not healthy, and who wishes to make changes. It is a fascinating, wise, thorough and potentially life-changing book.'

– Elizabeth Turp, NHS primary care counsellor and author of Chronic fatigue syndrome/ME: Support for Family and Friends

'This book has been written by a healthcare professional who has been through the chronic fatigue journey herself. It is aimed at both those going through the difficult journey of ME and the healthcare professionals working with those people. You can pick and choose your way across the chapters, choosing whichever needs or symptoms you want to understand and work with. Each chapter has focused exercises and summaries which mean you don't even necessarily have to read the entire chapter. From a healthcare professional's point of view, there are plenty of technical references to get your teeth into. I like the way the book also encompasses the mind/body connection as well as the more grounded physical aspects of working through chronic fatigue.'

– Laurel Alexander, author of How to Incorporate Wellness Coaching into Your Therapeutic Practice

'Lucie Montpetit's unique programme, laid out in this book, combines scientific research with principles from psychology to equip the reader with the knowledge and capacity to help themselves, and feel the positive impact of doing so.'

– Nicole Seguin, Clinical Psychologist, Montreal, Canada

BREAKING FREE FROM PERSISTENT FATIGUE

of related interest

Chronic Fatigue Syndrome/ME
Support for Family and Friends
Elizabeth Turp
Part of the Support for Family and Friends series
ISBN 978 1 84905 141 5
eISBN 978 0 85700 347 8

Body Intelligence
Creating a New Environment
2nd Edition
Ged Sumner
ISBN 978 1 84819 026 9
eISBN 978 0 85701 011 7

Managing Stress with Qigong
Gordon Faulkner
Foreword by Carole Bridge
ISBN 978 1 84819 035 1
eISBN 978 0 85701 016 2

Managing Depression with Qigong
Frances Gaik
ISBN 978 1 84819 018 4
eISBN 978 0 85701 006 3

Chair Yoga
Seated Exercises for Health and Wellbeing
Edeltraud Rohnfeld
Illustrated by Edeltraud Rohnfeld
Translated by Anne Oppenheimer
ISBN 978 1 84819 078 8
eISBN 978 0 85701 056 8

You Are How You Move
Experimental Chi Kung
Ged Sumner
ISBN 978 1 84819 014 6
eISBN 978 0 85701 002 5

Meet Your Body
CORE Bodywork and Rolfing Tools to Release Bodymindcore Trauma
Noah Karrasch
Illustrated by Lovella Lindsey
ISBN 978 1 84819 016 0
eISBN 978 0 85701 065 0

BREAKING FREE
FROM PERSISTENT FATIGUE

Lucie Montpetit

SINGING
DRAGON

LONDON AND PHILADELPHIA

Illustrations kindly provided by Genevieve April.
Table 1.1 on p.19 reproduced from Holmes and Rahe (1967) with kind permission from Elsevier.
Quotation on p.160 reproduced from Kübler-Ross (1969) with kind permission from the EKR Foundation.
Quotation on p.188 reproduced from McColl (2003) with kind permission from CAOT.
Quotation on p.199 reproduced from Townsend *et al.* (1991) with kind permission from CAOT.

First published in 2012
by Singing Dragon
an imprint of Jessica Kingsley Publishers
116 Pentonville Road
London N1 9JB, UK
and
400 Market Street, Suite 400
Philadelphia, PA 19106, USA

www.singingdragon.com

Library of Congress Cataloging in Publication Data
A CIP catalog record for this book is available from the Library of Congress

British Library Cataloguing in Publication Data
A CIP catalogue record for this book is available from the British Library

ISBN 978 1 84819 101 3
eISBN 978 0 85701 081 0

Printed and bound in Great Britain

Contents

Acknowledgements

I would first of all like to extend a 'super ultra mega' thank you to my sons, Daniel and Antoine. They were the catalysts who forced me to grow through adversity. Guys, thank you for your hugs, especially in the evening, when I was determined, even though I was exhausted, to read you stories; thank you for your amazing smiles every day, which are the best medicine in the world.

I also want to mention the precious help I received from several individuals: my mother Aline, as well as Huguette, Nela, Linda, Netti and François, who acted as an extension of my arms and legs at a time when I was in my worst shape. I want to extend a special thank you to my father for having taught me, during his own rehabilitation, determination and open-mindedness toward changes in habits; I'm sending love up in the direction of his star. And I would like to thank you, Richard, my long-time companion, for your confidence in my abilities, your wonderful open-mindedness, your 'non-judgement', your patience during some of those painful years, and your support in all aspects of our family life. Your love enabled me to overcome the hardship of the illness, redirect my career, and finish this book, while being surrounded by respect and tenderness.

I have to thank all the healthcare professionals who took the time to answer my questions so I could validate the foundations of my work. Such an inclusive perspective required me to delve into very specific pearls of wisdom. They answered my queries and, based on their areas of expertise, agreed to review certain sections of this book.

I wish to thank the homeopath Lynda Berthiaume, for sharing her understanding of the psycho-neuro-immuno-endocrine (PNI) super system, her remarkable professional skills, and her friendship. I would also like to acknowledge the clinical nutritionist Annick Lavoie, who effectively reopened her books to review sections of this manuscript that fell outside my area of professional expertise. This data was crucial to my understanding of the energy aspect of nutrients.

I need to mention Annemarie Couture, occupational therapist, who founded the centre *l'Essence en mouvement*, and who shared with me her expertise in sensory integration. Thank you, Francine Ferland, occupational therapy professor at the École de réadaptation at Université de Montréal, for her relevant feedback. I am so very thankful to Hélène Martel and Velda Lulic, osteopaths, for their support. Their theoretical knowledge of the body–mind was beyond invaluable to me.

As for Beatriz Padovan and her daughter, Dr Sonia Padovan-Catenne, who shared their passion and knowledge with me, where do I even start? These two women have put rehabilitation on the map and teach neurofunctional reorganization (the Padovan Method®) all over the world. This highly effective work tool has allowed me to regulate the autonomic nervous system of my most severely disabled patients.

I would like to express my appreciation to Dr Barry Breger, who followed and supported me throughout my own rehabilitation, tolerating my questions, my scepticism, and sometimes my stubbornness, before I would agree – or sometimes disagree – to follow his treatment recommendations. I would like to thank the acupuncturist Jacynthe Soucy, who used principles of Eastern medicine to answer my questions. I would also like to mention the remarkable work of the therapist Kyra Lober, who applies several techniques, including cranio-sacral therapy and Body–Mind Centering®. Kyra was able to relieve my constant pain and taught me some Oriental wisdom that made me a better therapist.

I am also grateful to a long-standing colleague and friend, psychologist Nicole Séguin, for her expertise, her opinions and her relevant suggestions on concepts falling outside of my comfort zone. On several occasions, Nicole encouraged me to get right back to work.

Finally, I would like to mention the work of Pamela Lipson, who made my text fluid in English, who took the time to understand the nuances of my writing, and who knew how to find just the right words to translate my colourful French-Canadian expressions. I would also like to thank Jasmine Petitclair, who provided the extensive computer support that this book required. Thank you to all the 'pseudo-normal' individuals, friends and acquaintances who responded to my list of energy-draining symptoms – which enabled me to put the finishing touches to the final version of this book.

Introduction

I have observed in my practice that exceptional patients, who share the responsibilities of their treatment with the health professionals surrounding them, feel empowered and get better faster.

It was on a sunny day back in March 2003 that my life started to turn upside down. I had gone to see my doctor because I was experiencing sudden energy lows, frequent drops in blood pressure, and food intolerances that worsened from week to week. In April 2003, due to a series of stressors that were attacking me from all angles, I discovered that I was suffering from an adjustment disorder.[1] Six months later, my doctor and I had no choice but to come to terms with the reality of the situation: the diagnosis was only partly correct. My pain was constant, my energy losses were becoming increasingly frequent, and would arise suddenly, and my strength and physical endurance were basically in a free fall. The diagnosis of an adjustment disorder implied that the psychosocial stressors that I had been dealing with for several months were at the root of my problems. That being said, in light of my medical history, we were forced to recognize that the symptoms had manifested themselves *before* the stressors appeared. With the physiological damage becoming more serious, a diagnosis was made: myalgic encephalomyelitis (also known as chronic fatigue immune dysfunction syndrome). Several weeks later, I was no longer able to adequately assume any of the roles I held in society. I needed other help from other people on a daily basis, I could no longer do my work as an occupational therapist, nor take care of the house. Sometimes, I couldn't even drive my car. I was bedridden all the time, except when I needed to take care of the kids early in the morning and after school, which demanded an enormous amount of effort on my part. Even if I had many projects in mind, and despite a passionate will to live that kept me going, I no longer had the strength I had once had to do the activities I once loved to engage in. I felt dispossessed; my body and my brain reacted in a fashion totally different from what I was accustomed to. My batteries were dead but I had no idea how to recharge them! I no longer knew how to swim, or even float and let myself drift along with the current. It's as if I had to fight to simply keep my head above water, and I no longer knew how to recover. The more I struggled, the more I lost the energy I needed to survive.

What was happening to me? What was the psychological reason (or reasons) for this fluctuation, followed by this almost total lack of energy? Pain, severe loss of cognitive skills, mental confusion, weakness, dizziness, lack of coordination, a burning sensation under the skin, the inability to make simple decisions, irritability... I didn't understand any of it! Driven by the need to know as much as by fear of the unknown, I began to comb through my medical science and occupational therapy books. I devoured scientific articles and research publications that addressed the symptoms I was exhibiting. As I had many cognitive deficits (trouble concentrating, memory lapses, and indecisiveness, etc.), I set out to produce summaries of the texts I was reading. I wrote in order to try to understand what was happening to me. It was a sort of therapeutic activity: rather than panicking and falling into a state of despondency – which would have led me straight into a depression – I was simply shifting my focus while acquiring valuable knowledge. I did not yet realize that I was writing for you, who are so tired, who do not understand the reason for such fatigue, and who are unable to cope.

This book provides concrete evidence. I have drawn on my personal experience and on my work performed on people suffering from various illnesses and from persistent fatigue as an incapacitating symptom. Here and there, I provide examples from personal and professional observations to support the theories and perspectives I am proposing. I am performing this exercise both from the point of view of a person who wants to heal and from that of a professional, namely, an occupational therapist. I tried to understand how a disciplined, energetic, athletic person in good health, with a zest for life, who watched her diet, could effectively harm her physiological, emotional, and cognitive system to the point of exhaustion. What was there to understand? The answers I found are based on known scientific facts and increasingly validated scientific hypotheses.

I wanted to give a name to this highly unrecognized, yet so currently widespread, health problem that could be considered a disease of the twenty-first century. I have to say, however, that after having exhibited the multitude of symptoms associated with the condition and having continued my research, speaking of a 'disease' seems inaccurate. The lack of energy and the various symptoms that are related to this problem have become almost commonplace – an everyday lot that falls to us, a sort of misery in this new century. The daily fatigue that is present from the time one wakes up until the moment one returns from work, this fatigue that seems normal to us because we believe it to be a by-product of work and of our many responsibilities, actually masks a physiological imbalance that could end up by producing a domino effect on our health. When fatigue becomes a daily symptom, it needs to be regarded as a warning sign. I will therefore refer to *energy imbalance* or *imbalance of the psycho-neuro-immuno-endocrine* (PNI) *system* as the syndrome that encompasses *persistent fatigue* and all the related symptoms.

To begin understanding this phenomenon, we will start by introducing the idea that adrenal fatigue could be one of the causes of an adjustment disorder – and of a *burnout*, which is one of the forms taken by an adjustment disorder – of which persistent fatigue is one of the consequences. We will then establish a connection with other illnesses in which the lack of energy and vitality is only the tip of the iceberg. This unorthodox overview is necessary. To go back to my personal situation, I should specify that far from ending with the last diagnosis, my journey was just beginning. On this journey, I was suffering from the following syndromes: myalgic encephalomyelitis (ME), also known as 'chronic fatigue syndrome' (CFS), and its cousin, fibromyalgia; multiple environmental sensitivities, food intolerances, allergies; leaky gut syndrome, dysbiosis, candidiasis (which traditional medicine does not yet recognize as a diagnosis); Costen's syndrome (known as temporo-mandibular joint dysfunction, or TMJD); and irritable bowel syndrome (IBS). Some of these problems are directly or indirectly related to persistent fatigue, partly based on individuals' genetic baggage and the environment in which they develop.

I will also point out all the auto-immune diseases that link back to persistent fatigue and energy imbalance and will address the issue of depression (primary or secondary) and anxiety disorders, whose symptoms often accompany the previously mentioned syndromes.

Ignoring the diagnoses for now, we will examine them through a different lens, by linking them to the phenomenon of allergies and all types of intolerances. We will discover that added to cancer (last century's demon) is an array of civilization-attacking evils (modern diseases) that seem to share many of the same features.

My healing process took two and a half years before I could regain my energy balance. In all humility, my goal is to make all this knowledge accessible to all those who, like me, have knocked on the doors of doctors and specialists, of healthcare professionals and alternative medicine advocates, only to come out empty-handed, finding no reasons for their dreaded afflictions. It was also important for me to address this book to occupational therapists, who are being increasingly solicited to work with people suffering from persistent fatigue, who must deal with the repercussions of the very real physical and psychological energy loss that brings their patients' daily activities to a screeching halt. We, as healthcare professionals, perceive this lack of energy in our patients as a symptom related to a psychological problem while all the cells in their body are screaming: 'Help! I need fuel!'

Regarding cancer, Dr Siegel has claimed that when people are given the choice between surgery and a lifestyle change, eight out of ten people choose the operation![2] Out of five people who seek to achieve a state of well-being by beating this common problem of persistent fatigue, I can therefore conclude that I get through to at least one of them. It's a very good start! But I also know that many people do not immediately find the courage to implement changes in their lives. Although this is a possibility that exists for every one of us, adjusting habits is not something that everyone can easily accept, or even imagine. I nevertheless believe that we shouldn't wait until we are forced to finally take action, or until we are no longer able to carry out our daily responsibilities, or until we go through the turmoil I went through that pushed me to take charge of my life and initiate a healing process. And when we are well equipped and ready, we need to find the strength necessary to break free from denial and leave our former beliefs behind. This strength lies within us, not in a book.

I have learned a lot through observing many patients, especially those suffering from auto-immune, neurological, and degenerative diseases. The most fulfilled were beaming with courage, open-mindedness and hope.

I sincerely think that many people diagnosed as *chronic* have not yet reached the point of no return; I observe it among the rest of the patients in my practice. I believe that the word 'chronic' should not be associated with any diagnosis because it acts as a *nocebo* (negative placebo) and can lead the person, and the people in their life (including healthcare professionals), to lose sight of the one thing they so imperatively require to improve their situation: *hope*.

This book is a guide intended to help you to embark on a personal journey. On this journey, you will discover that it is possible to become increasingly in control of your body–mind. In turn, this body–mind will guide you because you will have learned how to decipher it. This book is a tool that will help you to draw up a sort of balance sheet of your energy state – as you would do if your financial position was suffering. You will then be better able to make concrete changes to your habits and verify that these changes are in fact effective. It is also a guide for healthcare professionals, particularly for occupational therapists treating clients suffering from persistent fatigue. These professionals will find tools that will enable them to assist the patients who are too cognitively impaired to read this book.

If you are very tired, overstressed, exhausted, or on the road to becoming so, if you feel voided at the least physical effort or after exerting the least amount of effort, if you are at the end of your rope, at the point of being incapable of working or of shouldering your family and personal responsibilities, if you want to understand a little more about what is happening to you and if you are interested in getting better, I recommend this book. It will help you to rise to the challenge which, I realize, is enormous, but which, believe me, is worth the effort. Those people in whom a state of deterioration has led to an auto-immune or degenerative disease will perhaps find ways of alleviating their suffering and of improving their quality of life; they will know on what door to knock to find help, and even to mitigate their symptoms and delay regression. And, who knows, they might even learn how to heal the inner malaise and grow while tackling the illness head on. Turn the page. A hot sun will warm you little by little, as long as you are ready to free yourself from the belief that it does not exist when the clouds stand in the way…

It is a fact that modern medicine is wonderful for its competence in emergency situations. However, too many patients feel disappointed with the medical approach to modern diseases related to stress.

How to Use this Book

The chapters in this book are designed for you to be able to consult them based on your expectations. Each chapter will guide you to other chapters that will be able to answer your various questions. Let your needs guide you while you read this book. If, for example, you are at a stage where you feel highly exhausted and have trouble concentrating, I suggest that you go directly to the chapters that provide advice on 'how to survive on little energy' so you can rebuild yourself from a physiological standpoint (particularly Chapters 4 and 5). Most of the chapters are designed to enable you to directly consult (at the end of the chapter) the exercises to do or the summaries that, in order to save energy, you may prefer to read first. You can always refer to the theoretical explanations later when your energy and concentration levels improve. You cannot avoid reading Chapter 3, and doing the proposed exercises if you are going to complete your energy balance sheet. You can then move on to the habit-modifying exercises in Chapters 8 to 11. When you need to carry one of the Appendices around with you to refer to, you can download and print a copy from www.jkp.com/catalogue/book/9781848191013/resources.

And no, you don't need to do all the exercises in this book! There is more than one way to improve your health. Choose the tools to which you can relate. We don't all waste our energy for the same reasons, or in the same way, for that matter. Each person has genetic and environmental baggage that is specific to them. Each person has a belief system in which the relationship between energizing and energy-draining sources is perceived differently. If you prefer to read this book from cover to cover, make sure you have the energy required to do so. And again, use only the exercises that are relevant for you.

Certain specifications and references have been added, intended for those who require a scientific explanation, as well as for healthcare professionals who wish to gain a better grasp of the complexity of certain problems from which their clients are suffering. These references and specifications are not required for vitality to be recovered or for the inner journey to occur, however they will enable a person to make sound choices regarding their state of health and remain active in the decision-making process with respect to the recommended therapy.

Some people will need guidance and help from a healthcare professional during the various steps of the process. As the reality of today's depleted healthcare system offers us no more than a few minutes to explain our problems to a physician, it is essential to arrive well prepared, with a list of questions and observations. I have therefore included in this book some tools that I have presented in the form of charts and rating scales, in an effort to facilitate access to relevant information, both for the reader and the healthcare professional.

I wrote this book because I believe that each one of us is largely responsible for the journey we take, for our health, and for our inner well-being, on a daily basis. To test this theory, I can assure you that the following advice is justified: 'Ask, and it shall be given you; seek, and ye shall find; knock, and it shall be opened for you: for every one that asketh receiveth; and he that seeketh, findeth; and to him that knocketh it shall be opened.'[1] It's a matter of being honest, of opening your eyes, of getting rid of the blinkers, and of being attentive. To search is to embark on a process along which answers will come to us. The answer we receive is not always what we are expecting, but it helps us to grow nonetheless... May this book help you on this journey.

Chapter 1

What Is this Fatigue that Never Seems to End?

Chaos: A condition of great disorder or confusion.

Equilibrium: A condition in which all acting influences are cancelled by others, resulting in a stable, balanced system.

We spend energy every single moment of our lives. Even when we are not moving, we spend energy to think. And if we had enough discipline not to think, even just for a few moments, we would still spend energy, that is, the energy required to sustain ourselves. The heart beats, breathing occurs, and the body temperature adjusts automatically. French physiologist Claude Bernard was the first to define this state of internal dynamic equilibrium that is achieved unconsciously and constantly within the body as *homeostasis*.

In reality, the only thing that does not change is change itself. And change requires that we adapt and adapting in turn generates stress. The more we have to adapt to change, whether it be physical, emotional, cognitive, sociocultural, or spiritual, the more we spend energy. The main message of this book will therefore not be that of avoiding change and stress – that would mean denying the fact that life is in a state of perpetual change – but rather to propose methods that will enable you to stop resisting and ride the wave of change and embrace its energy to cheerfully go wherever life takes you. What happens to us is neither good nor bad. It is simply life that comes with its ups and downs, its ambushes and its wonderful moments of joy, its gifts and its shortcomings. Life is defined by all these changes, so why deny them and dwell on the illusion of permanence? The wake-up call would only be that much more violent.

People who suffer from *persistent fatigue* have often had to deal with many major (good or bad) physical and/or psychosocial changes within a short period of time, hence the often proposed diagnosis of an adjustment disorder. We will begin our understanding with this classic explanation.

In the 1960s, Holmes and Rahe developed the Social Readjustment Rating Scale based on this hypothesis. Those researchers included 43 events to which the ratings were based on the degree of adaptation required (see Table 1.1). Even though this list is neither very up to date nor exhaustive, it at least provides us with a good starting point for understanding what is going on. The word *change* often reappears as a criterion on this scale. According to the authors, people with a result below 150 feel only minor stress; between 150 and 199, they experience mild stress, between 200 and 299, moderate stress; and over 300, they feel severe stress that leads to a serious illness or an accident in 80 per cent of cases.[1]

It is not exclusively the event itself that is stressful, but similarly all the small daily disruptions that result from the act of adjusting to this new challenge. For example, if you change jobs, you need to adapt to a new work schedule, to another itinerary and other travel conditions, and to learning about the different environment (new work colleagues, names to learn, specific procedures, the premises). All these new habits are intricately related to learning and developing new motor patterns. Perhaps there will also be adjustments related to the family schedule, and other adjustments related to the perception you have of your new job. Many small changes arise as a result of a single striking event. As such, in this context, we initially spend a lot of energy to acquire learning loops which, later on, will become automatic and efficient actions. They will simply become second nature.

TABLE 1.1 Social Readjustment Rating Scale[2]

RANK	LIFE EVENTS	LIFE CHANGE UNITS
1	Death of a spouse	100
2	Divorce	73
3	Marital separation	65
4	Jail term	63
5	Death of close family member	63
6	Personal injury or illness	53
7	Marriage	50
8	Fired from work	47
9	Marital reconciliation	45
10	Retirement	45
11	Change in health of family member	44
12	Pregnancy	40
13	Sexual difficulties	40
14	Gain of new family member	39
15	Major business readjustment	39
16	Change in financial state	38
17	Death of a close friend	37
18	Moving to a different line of work	36
19	Change in number of arguments with spouse	35
20	Taking on a new mortgage	31
21	Mortgage over $10000[1]	30
22	Change in responsibilities at work	29
23	Son/daughter leaving home	29
24	Problems with in-laws	29
25	Outstanding personal achievement	28
26	Wife[2] begins or stops work	26
27	Begin or end school	26
28	Change in living conditions	25
29	Change of personal habits	24
30	Problems with boss	23
31	Change in working hours or conditions	20
32	Change in residence	20
33	Change in schools	20
34	Change in recreation	19

RANK	LIFE EVENTS	LIFE CHANGE UNITS
35	Change in church activities	19
36	Change in social activities	18
37	Mortgage or loan less than $10000[3]	17
38	Change in sleeping habits	16
39	Change in number of family get-togethers	15
40	Change in eating habits	15
41	Vacation	13
	TOTAL	

1. Since the scale was created in 1967, this amount does not reflect present-day realities so consider reading instead: 'a major loan such as for the purchase of a house'.

2. Substitute 'Spouse' for 'Wife'.

3. Small mortgage or loan such as for home renovations or the purchase of a car.

List of symptoms

You are more irritable than usual. The sound of the radio, the neighbour's barking dog, the shouts of children playing…all put a real strain on you. You suffer from insomnia, or you wake up feeling tired after a long night's sleep. Your brain cannot be aroused after two or three espressos. In the evening, you may be accustomed to having a beer or a glass of wine to relax. You crash in front of the TV after supper; you doze off in your chair, or at the wheel, after a big meal with friends. Instead of feeling invigorated after a trip to the gym, you feel drained. You forget your keys, your wallet, your appointments. Your brain has been functioning in multitask mode for several months now; you are both tired and wired at the same time. You feel as if you are missing out on the little, everyday pleasures. Everything becomes a task, a burden…

Your perspiration smells more foul than usual. You feel dizzy when you take a shower or a hot bath, or when you get out of bed too quickly. You binge. Ladies, you experience hot flashes; you suffer from such a miserable premenstrual syndrome that your work colleagues, your spouse and your children avoid speaking to you the week before your period which is, by the way, very painful and abnormally heavy. Your menstrual cycle fluctuates or is shorter than it was in the past, even though you are hardly approaching menopause. Your sex drive is nonexistent or exacerbated. Men, your libido is flat and your sexual performance sometimes falls flat. 'But what is happening to me?' you ask yourself. Basically, you no longer recognize yourself.

The list of symptoms in Tables 1.2 and 1.3 will provide you with some tips if you are suffering from a syndrome of which one of the major symptoms is persistent fatigue. It's possible that you have been downplaying these signs or that you are unaware of them. Take the time to read this table that lists the symptoms of energy exhaustion. Observe yourself three times over several days, refer to the questionnaire and record your results in the three columns. Don't look for problems where they don't exist. This range of symptoms includes several forms of different manifestations that result in an energy imbalance. You certainly do not suffer from all of these aches and pains and of those from which you do suffer, some seem to come and go. Be as honest with yourself as possible. These symptoms are messages that your body is sending you and that you should learn how to decipher, and not take simply as the issuance of a harsh sentence.

Total the results and check the changes after 8 to 12 weeks in order to objectify your condition. This test has not been standardized, but it gives a good idea of the state of health or of the extent of the psycho-neuro-immuno-endocrine (PNI) imbalance. It is also a good tool to use for presenting your symptoms to your family doctor in a quick and organized fashion.[3]

What causes these different symptoms? Is there or is there not a common trigger? Is it something that stems from a post-infection syndrome, a parasite, a pollution effect, a psychosocial stress, a dietary deficiency, a lifestyle effect, genetics, or a little of all of the above? Some symptoms are diffused and, at first glance, do not seem to be interrelated. Could they be variations on the same theme? Science is just beginning to (only partially) answer these questions. In Chapter 13, you will find a brief overview of the hormonal imbalance that causes some of these symptoms.

Stress stems from various sources. Based on each person's genetics, stressors or often normal and inevitable life changes – an infection, a parasite, abuse, an accident or a disease from which one has suffered – will accentuate the weaknesses of a more sensitive organ or of an aspect of the physiological system. We will try to understand some of the functions of this system by referring to the *PNI model*. This paradigm is drawing a rising number of supporters in the medical world because it is more complete than the traditional model.

TABLE 1.2 List of energy-draining symptoms: PNI imbalance syndrome

KEY TO SCORING:

Never	Rarely (1x/month)	Sometimes (2 to 4x/month)	Often (More than 1x/week)	Every day
0	1	2	3	4

PHYSICAL MANIFESTATIONS	DATE:		
1. I have dry eyes			
2. My mouth is dry			
3. I suffer from migraines			
4. I suffer from headaches			
5. I suffer from sleep disorders			
6. I experience dizziness or vertigo			
7. I feel nauseous or sick to my stomach without any apparent reason			
8. I am hypersensitive to noise			
9. I am hypersensitive to light			
10. I am hypersensitive to odours			
11. My eyes are irritated			
12. I get hives			
13. I feel itchy			
14. I have palpitations			
15. I am short of breath			
16. I feel cold			
17. My hands and/or my feet are cold			
18. At rest, my hands are warm and sweaty			
19. *I lose my hair more than normal (*Score: 0 or 4*)			
20. I have chest pain			
21. I am intolerant to cold			
22. I get tremors when I am under pressure or tired			
23. I get tremors when I am at rest: hands, tongue, or eyelids			
24. I get inner tremors			
25. I suffer from involuntary movements of the arms and/or legs			
26. My ankles swell at night			
27. When I scratch myself, a white line appears on my skin for a few minutes			
28. *I have developed brown spots on my face, neck or shoulders (*Score: 0 or 4*)			
29. *I have gained weight in the abdominal area (*Score: 0 or 4*)			
30. I have food cravings: starch, sweet desserts			
31. I have salt cravings			

32. I suffer from sudden energy drops			
33. I feel tired when I wake up, even after a good night's sleep			
34. My energy level drops around 10–11 am and/or 4 pm			
35. I get an energy boost in the evening			
36. I recently fainted			
37. I need to wake up to urinate 3 to 5 times a night			
38. I get dizzy from going from a reclining to a sitting position			
39. I get dizzy from going from a sitting to a standing position			
40. I feel agitated			
41. I do not tolerate physical exercise			
42. My muscles ache			
43. I have muscle cramps in the evening or during the night			
44. My joints ache			
45. I experience muscle weakness			
46. I tend to drop objects			
47. I do not digest well: bloating, burning, diarrhoea, constipation			
48. *I eat a lot but do not gain weight (Score: 0 or 4)			
49. The lymph nodes in my neck are swollen			
50. The lymph nodes in my armpits are swollen			
51. *I develop respiratory infections easily: cold, flu, bronchitis… (Score: 0 or 4)			
52. *The allergies and/or intolerances I suffer from are getting worse (Score: 0 or 4)			
53. I experience hot flushes at night			
54. My sex drive has increased			
55. My sex drive has decreased			
WOMEN (DO NOT COMPLETE IF YOU ARE POST-MENOPAUSAL)			
56. *I experience heavy bleeding and painful menstrual cramps (Score: 0 or 4)			
57. *My menstrual cycle fluctuates or is shorter than it used to be (Score: 0 or 4)			
58. *I experience one or two migraines per menstrual cycle (Score: 0 or 4)			
59. Sexual intercourse tires me out			
MEN			
56. I have trouble maintaining my erection			
57. Sexual intercourse tires me out more than usual			
TOTAL OUT OF 232 FOR WOMEN (220 AFTER MENOPAUSE) AND OUT OF 228 FOR MEN			

TABLE 1.3 Psycho-affective and psycho-cognitive manifestations

KEY TO SCORING:

Never	Rarely (1x/month)	Sometimes (2 to 4x/month)	Often (More than 1x/week)	Every day
0	1	2	3	4

PSYCHO-AFFECTIVE MANIFESTATIONS	DATE:		
1. I am irritable			
2. I do not tolerate stress			
3. I have unexplained fears and anxieties			
4. I avoid emotionally charged situations			
5. I need to rest after feeling tense or being emotional			
6. I feel depressed			
7. I feel both tired and agitated			
8. I feel frustrated			
9. I have mood swings			
10. I feel guilty			
11. I feel anxious during the night			
12. I suffer from panic attacks			
TOTAL OUT OF 48			
PSYCHO-COGNITIVE MANIFESTATIONS			
1. I have trouble concentrating			
2. I frequently forget little things: my keys, something in the house, an appointment…			
3. I do not think clearly			
4. I have memory problems			
5. I have trouble making up my mind			
6. I am increasingly disorganized in my work environment, in my thoughts, at home, in my family life…			
7. I find myself searching for my words and forgetting them			
8. I feel confused intellectually when I am under pressure, in a hurry or when I am emotional			
9. I am disorganized			
10. I lack initiative			
11. I no longer take the initiative to do the activities I used to engage in			
12. I have recurring thoughts in my head that I have trouble getting rid of			
13. I am not as productive as I was a year ago (or as I was before my disease started)			
TOTAL OUT OF 52			
TOTAL (AFFECTIVE + COGNITIVE) OUT OF 100			

Is it normal to have an abnormal stress rate?

...in terms of mortality, stress poses a more
serious risk factor than tobacco.[4]

Let's remember that stress is a normal and desirable phenomenon in many situations. The famous 'fight or flight'[5] principle reminds us of this. And even when we do not flee or fight when confronted with danger, but when we still need to be on the defensive, stress is what helps to stimulate our vigilance. Stress is part of every situation in which there is a new challenge to face. It's part of our daily lives. It's our body–mind's reaction to any change. Change is simply a part of life. If nothing changes, there is stagnation, and that would mean life no longer exists. Without feeling or perhaps realizing it, we are constantly changing to maintain our body's *homeostasis*. It would therefore be ludicrous to say that to live better we should strive to avoid change or stress.

So where does the problem lie? A part of our brain, known as *autonomous* or *primitive*, is designed perfectly to address this type of situation – for example, in the bush, an animal starts running to escape the wildcat. But how do we react when the so-called wildcat is a vehicle that cuts in front of us on the road and we are enclosed in our car?

The adrenal glands are perceived as being the first to show signs of fatigue for the simple reason that they have the greatest amount of work to get done in terms of self-protective functions, as you will see in Chapter 13. In the 1950s, in Montreal, Dr Hans Selye conducted extensive research on stress in rats. He admirably described the *General Adaptation Syndrome* (GAS) to stress.[6] He described the effects of stressors on rats, leading to the destruction of the *adrenal glands* (endocrine system), the cerebral *hippocampus* (nervous system), and especially the spectacular atrophy of the *thymus* (immune system).[7] In a single day, after having subjected the rats to a trauma or a sudden illness, Selye explains that millions of immune system cells, called lymphocytes, were destroyed and that the volume of their thymus had decreased by half! How is it that we pay so little attention to such specific studies conducted in rats, while the stressors and effects undergone are so accurately supported by the type of stress and signs that we are currently coming up against in the twenty-first century?

Since the findings on intolerances and food allergies (immune system),[8] we could have thought that these old problems, which are nevertheless increasingly frequent, were going to be considered by modern medicine. But still too often, modern medicine only treats the symptoms, without focusing on the causes.

The overstress on the adrenal glands, described by Dr Wilson, is not considered a medical diagnosis. Unless an individual suffers from Addison's disease, which is an extreme form of adrenal insufficiency, blood tests are not designed to adequately screen out the adrenal insufficiency that would follow the testing of multiple stressors. In medicine, adrenal insufficiency is only considered when it results from the absorption of an excessive dose of steroids (as a legal drug or not).[9] We are only just beginning to consider that a cascade of stressors leading to an excessive production of *cortisol* – the stress hormone – could yield the same results. You can refer to a summary of the functions of cortisol in a stressful situation in Chapter 13.

In medicine, urine and blood analyses use standards that are considered as being representative of the average population. However, and even though *adrenal insufficiency* is not screened out by these analyses, most North Americans suffer from adrenal insufficiency at one point or another or suffer from it on a daily basis without even knowing it. Can one seriously regard as normal these symptoms that fail to screen out *adrenal fatigue* in a society afflicted by stressors that are multiplying at a feverish rate? According to Dr Wilson, close to 67 per cent of the American population would be afflicted with moderate to severe adrenal fatigue![10] In 2002, Dr John Stewart estimated that hydrostatic hypertension, one of the causes of which is adrenal insufficiency, had a prevalence of 7 to 30 per cent among older people and was underdiagnosed.[11]

One of the reasons why receiving adequate diagnosis and treatment is so difficult is due to the fact that medical training is based on a specialization model. Consequently, it is difficult to find a physician who analyses hormonal results from a general perspective, that is, relating some results with others and in relation to the rates of certain minerals such as, for example, magnesium, which is very instrumental in the production of intracellular energy. Some physicians will be sensitive to hypoglycaemic symptoms, but when the blood sugar or urine tests yield average results, they don't push their investigation any further.

Doctor, what is the diagnosis?

One of the most widespread diseases is 'diagnosis'.[12]

Karl Kraus

In order to better understand the symptomatology of Table 1.2 I have created Appendix 1, which will make it possible to compare symptoms. I have included symptoms from several diagnoses related to persistent fatigue. In Appendix 2 I compare most of these symptoms with the effects caused by mineral and vitamin nutritional deficiencies.

What struck me while I was compiling Appendix 1 was the complexity of the relationships between the different body–mind systems and the obvious similarities between the symptoms among the different diagnoses. It is as if the diagnosis could differ depending on the specialist who is examining you, and according to the way in which you describe your symptoms. It is therefore important to provide you with good tools in order to be effectively heard by your physician. You can easily find yourself with a wrong diagnosis or even, as in my case, without a diagnosis, until you reach the point at which the elastic snaps. This was what pushed me to develop the list of symptoms in Tables 1.2 and 1.3.

To gain an understanding of the complexity of the symptomatology, I had to change my way of understanding disease in general – the way I had been taught in university. The paradigm that I had learned needed to be improved. Once the perspective is adjusted to accommodate a more comprehensive overview, it becomes possible to better situate the various proposed diagnoses.

Adrenal fatigue is too restrictive a diagnosis because even though the adrenal glands are perhaps the first to release signs of distress, it is the entire endocrine system that is in a state of imbalance. *Hypoglycaemia* may be as much of a consequence as it is a cause of an imbalance. *Neuroendocrine exhaustion* also does not take into account the complete reality of the syndrome because the immune system components are not reflected, and once they are in a state of imbalance, these systems lead to all sorts of other illnesses, especially auto-immune ones, which are more specific to each person's genetic makeup: rheumatoid arthritis, lupus erythematosus, Hashimoto's disease, diabetes, multiple sclerosis, certain cardiac conditions… And by their very nature, these conditions further offset the PNI system.

And even if in a situation of acute stress you undergo routine blood tests, it is likely that the results will remain within the limits of normality, as the norms have been so extensively broadened. As such, you could see your exhaustion fall under the heading of *hypochondria*, as the symptoms are neither specifically applied to an organ, nor do they demonstrate a disease according to accepted standards.[13] I suspect, however, that in the twenty-first century, the standard does not correspond with normality, that it only reflects an average in which the trend is itself maintained in a state of abnormality. The designation of *chronic fatigue syndrome* bothers me because the word *chronic* connotes the idea of a sentencing to remain ill. Word choice is very important if one's intention is to suggest a return to a healthy state, a hope for something better.

It is clear that *psychological distress* often shares a link with this body–mind disharmony. Also, *reactional depression* may be included among all the perverse secondary effects of energy exhaustion. But it cannot be accepted as the primary diagnosis for all forms of exhaustion, for this would be mainly to take into account the mental symptoms while, in reality, one struggles with many physiological symptoms, which are not adequately considered or which are dissociated from cognitive and emotional difficulties.

An adjustment disorder is seen as a reaction that is poorly adapted to an identifiable psychosocial stressor, but the society in which we live pushes us, by virtue of the beliefs it conveys – productivity, performance, and hyperconsumption – to exceed our possibilities of adapting, at many levels. We increasingly try to adapt to an unbalanced environment. By definition, an adjustment disorder lasts a maximum of six months. But, given that the reality of our feverish pace and the resulting abnormality are perpetuated in our environment, medicine must find, once the six months are up, another epithet.

Some people who are weakened by persistent fatigue often suffer from ailments related to the physical environment, whether it be multiple chemical sensitivity (MCS), any type of allergy, food intolerance, or even irritable bowel syndrome.[14]

In the twenty-first century the Western medical model still exists and persists in our health system. Although it is still valid, a part of the scientific community is currently giving it special treatment by including it in a new paradigm in which the interrelationship between the systems of the human body is regarded without the fixed hierarchy that was once assigned to it. As such, the advent of a new medical paradigm shows us that all these illnesses share a common thread: a too easily alarmed inflammatory process, hence the possibility of a disrupted immune system. This is what leads us to once again address the PNI system in which all the systems are intimately interrelated. The *psycho-neuro-immuno-endocrine imbalance* (which I will refer to as 'PNI imbalance') thus gives expression, in my opinion, to these illnesses from which our society so frequently suffers.

To understand this broad-spectrum model, we are going to explore Selye's General Adaptation Syndrome. This will give us, by the same token, an overview of what happens to us before general and persistent exhaustion is manifested. In my opinion, it's like starting a puzzle by selecting the pieces of the framework in order to be able to more easily structure the whole.

General Adaptation Syndrome (GAS)

Every stress leaves a scar and speeds up the ageing process.

Dr Selye defines GAS in three stages: the alarm reaction, the stage of resistance, and the stage of exhaustion.[15] To describe these phases, I will compare our PNI system with an energy bank – if we put energy on the same plane as money, we can always earn more once we have landed the right job or when we apply a sound financial strategy. Although vital energy can feed on energizing nourishment in all aspects of human activity and can prosper according to our mental ability to produce results, its production is limited by our genetic baggage and the proper functioning of the systems responsible for its production and use of energy. From a financial standpoint, we can change jobs for something more lucrative, but from a physiological perspective, we cannot change our glands and cellular makeup to produce more energy once we have optimized their performance.

Basic level of resistance

At this level, we deposit our paycheque regularly (in all respects: physical, emotional, mental, sociocultural, and spiritual) and we withdraw money to cover the costs related to our daily needs. There is a balance between what goes in and what comes out.

By taking care of my body through healthy nutrition, moderate physical exercise, by ensuring a balance between my responsibilities and my leisure activities, and by performing my daily activities with a light-hearted attitude, I am figuratively depositing money into my account mind by the way in which I approach my daily life, the situations that arise and the people I deal with. I feel good about the little pleasures in my life: it's a good investment for the future. My entire endocrine system is in harmony with the other systemic components of my body – everything is for the best.

Alarm reaction

When something unexpected occurs, such as a physical or mental shock, exposure to environmental pollutants or a combination of several of these stressors, I enter the alarm stage. I temporarily mortgage my house (my body–mind) to take care of some urgent renovation work. Hepatic functions are decreased.[16] My endocrine system is highly solicited: it must be able to produce more hormones so I can accommodate the demand for the additional energy I require. I then decrease the functions that are not essential for immediate survival (digestion) and I supply more energy to my muscles to be able to *fight or flee*. Although there is no big bad wolf clawing at my heels, my body reacts as if I were in this type of survival situation. By stepping up my energy spending in this way, I create more waste and my immune system has to work harder to take care of this additional waste.

I spend more than I earn. I have fewer opportunities to put money away in my pension fund. In the case of a rat, the adrenal glands (endocrine system) swell and the thymus (immune system) shrinks.[17]

Recovery stage

Everything quickly returns to its original state if the problem is easily resolved and if it is short lived. I restore my body–mind with adequate rest and quality food. I pay what I owe and I replenish my pension fund.

Stage of resistance

It can also happen that I find myself faced with a new warning. If it temporarily appears on the scene and quickly disappears, a new recovery stage, sometimes one that takes a little longer, will follow. When the problem persists and other problems arise, I shift from the alarm stage into the resistance stage. I adapt to my standard of living. I don't necessarily oppose, I don't flee, but I am on the lookout for potential danger. I am on my guard. I am vigilant. With time, my perception becomes coloured by apprehension, which further consumes my energy.

I work overtime to pay off my energy mortgage and I apply for a line of credit to maintain my lifestyle. From a physiological perspective, my endocrine glands, particularly my adrenal glands and my pancreas which works with my liver, are highly solicited to produce energy from glucose and to balance this glucose level. The pancreas also works to produce enzymes in order to allow the nutrients required to produce this energy to be absorbed: this production will possibly decline if it is no longer effectively synchronized with the digestive rhythms that are unbalanced by stress or if the pancreas weakens. My body evacuates toxins by working overtime (transpiration, bile salts, lymphatic and digestive systems' excretion). I realize that something is not quite right, but I am not changing anything in my approach. Since I am prepared to fight, my body also secretes endorphins to help me to tolerate pain: the resistance ensures that I do not feel signs of any disturbance.

If the situation worsens and I continue to adapt, my vigilance becomes constant. I avoid spending unnecessarily to save my money for emergency expenses. Because of my hypervigilance, I have the impression that I am being assaulted from all angles. I have less and less time for leisure activities and I seem to be incapable of returning to where I was prior to entering the alarm stage. Although the stress hormone, cortisol, is always assessed within normal limits in the blood, it is higher than it was in the past. Insulin continues to facilitate the penetration of glucose into my cells. In certain people, a disruption occurs and glucose no longer adequately penetrates the cells. This resistance of the cells to glucose causes greater fatigue. One must realize that the brain is particularly vulnerable to the lack of glucose required for survival and for the nervous cells to function properly: intolerance to noise, impatience, trouble concentrating, and the loss of short-term memory are neurological signs that should be cause for concern – but they occur in an insidious fashion: slowly and we adapt.

The hypothalamus remains constantly on guard. I am *tired and wired* at the same time. Stress becomes chronic. My creditors never leave me alone; I have trouble sleeping, my digestion is affected, I suffer from heartburn, diarrhoea and/or constipation, cognitive impairment, hypoglycaemia. The least intrusion and my body deploys its defence, setting off a highly charged inflammatory process which, based on each person's genetics, triggers migraines, more frequent respiratory and/or food allergies, back pain... I become more prone to infections; I catch colds more frequently, for example. Any inflammatory process will require an anti-inflammatory process, so an even greater secretion of cortisol by the adrenal glands! However, although cortisol has helped us to survive admirably for millennia, it becomes toxic for the brain when it is produced in too great a quantity... The vicious circle continues.

To produce cortisol, the endocrine system works overtime. The *circadian* hormonal secretion cycle becomes disrupted (see Chapter 7). The production of sexual hormones is sometimes thrown off balance to assist in this cortisol production. This imbalance can occur as much in the feminine as in the masculine gonads (heightened PMS, premature ejaculation, menstrual cycle without ovulation). The libido declines: in times of fighting, it is no time to think about having sex! The thyroid gland is also primed to be a contributor: it speeds up the metabolism to withdraw more energy from the system. It influences all the cells of the body–mind. Hyperventilating becomes a symptom. Some people undergo panic attacks.

The PNI imbalance helps to accentuate the survival reaction in the face of the least change because the body has more and more trouble maintaining its basic homeostatic balance. I avoid my creditors, not really knowing how to get myself out of this budgetary impasse. I drop my investments; I eat into my retirement savings to pay off debts that keep piling up, however...

Stage of exhaustion

...the cheques bounce and I pay surcharge fees. I don't manage to get ahead because interest charges eat into my meagre savings. Without capital, I am unable to pay off my debts. I don't even have the means to cover the basic daily expenses. I am in an exhaustion stage! Damage has occurred on a cellular level. I need to take a break from my activities to be able to use the energy required to help my body regenerate and repair the damage. But I have been sinking into debt for so long... I have lost my body's dynamic balance. The rate of blood cortisol perhaps falls within normal limits, but very close to the lower limit, while the rate of salivary cortisol is often low at certain times of the day.

Saliva hormone testing

In research, saliva testing is often used to determine hormone concentration. These tests are more sensitive than blood tests in this context. After failing to understand my state for four months, I decided to take a saliva hormone test to establish the rate of cortisol – the stress hormone – at four specific times of the day and at a specific point in my menstrual cycle based on an established protocol.[18] The tests revealed an abnormally low rate of salivary cortisol in the morning. The three other results were at the low end of average range.[19]

Two possibilities
Bankruptcy

An insidious inflammatory process gets underway more or less long term, according to each individual's genetic weaknesses. The exhausted body is possibly struggling with a more acidic environment and, as a result, becomes host to parasites that exacerbate the inflammatory process. Food intolerances and environmental sensitivities multiply, while symptoms of auto-immune diseases appear in people who are at higher risk.[20]

The production of endorphins declines and I start feeling pain that I didn't feel before because I was too focused on surviving. The pain itself can become energy-draining.

Conserving one's energy capital

It's time to take stock and gain an overview of your indebtedness. It's also important to meet with an advisor to consolidate the debts as required by your situation. If you don't take this step, the repercussions could prove disastrous and could lead you to bankruptcy.

The field of occupational therapy is commonly used to balance the energy demands on arthritic hands, or on the body of someone living with multiple sclerosis, or who has just undergone heart surgery. We try to make sure that patients have the tools to better manage their energy level on a daily basis, in the same way that your financial advisor would give you advice on how to slightly reduce the taxes you have to pay, make a guaranteed investment, and conserve your capital base as much as possible. If you are left with 40 per cent of your energy or financial capital, it is important to know what bills need to be paid first (tasks that absolutely need to be taken care of) and what investments (rest periods amidst calm and pleasure) and comforts (leisure and other activities) you can indulge in.

In Chapter 3 you will be invited to draw up a list of your daily activities and to evaluate their impact by becoming aware of how you perceive these activities. It is only when you have achieved this awareness that you will be able to apply, with a certain degree of effectiveness, the energy conservation methods with respect to organizing, planning, and making the decision to give priority to activities, and then simplify them. In Chapter 4, you will then acquire the tools to observe, on a monthly basis, the fluctuation in your daily energy level and the variables that cause this energy level to fluctuate.

In my university training, I learned various energy-management methods for patients suffering from incapacitating illnesses and whose lack of energy was a daily challenge. The methods used focus especially on habits:

- changes in behaviour based on the limitations of the disease

- ergonomic changes to work and home environments

- organization of work and other activities (including popular time management techniques).

However, my profession always proved useful when it came to addressing the client's limits and not their potential to recharge their batteries and rediscover a better functional level. There was one issue related to these energy-conservation and time-management techniques that I knew, namely, that of the cognitive symptoms and their repercussions.

Fragile body–mind homeostasis

The advice regarding energy conservation, of which I was aware, helped to limit the waste caused by the damage to my health but this advice was insufficient in helping me to recover and restore my health. Once I exerted the least physical effort, I had trouble maintaining my body–mind's homeostasis. I even had to avoid extreme heat in the summer and extreme cold in the winter: such conditions demanded too much energy of me.

Given that the organizational and planning capacity from a cerebral perspective is mortgaged, I sincerely believe that as long as the cognitive symptoms are incapacitating, it is useless to force yourself to plan and organize better. How do you go about organizing when you have become indecisive, when you tend to forget things easily, and when you are constantly searching for your words? You only need to take a look at your office, fridge, and bedroom to see that the lack of organization in your brain is projected onto your everyday life. My approach changed when I noticed this type of phenomenon. And it's this new approach that I am currently proposing.

Brain functioning and energy level

To my great astonishment, I once again became efficient and more orderly when the cognitive symptoms faded, and this occurred gradually as my energy level improved. This gradual process is parallel to the physiological energy level.

After having observed this phenomenon in several people, I am certain that energy conservation undergoes a process of reestablishing homeostasis and the physiological functions related to the primitive brain. In this way, the brain is more available for its expression, learning, and creativity functions, rather than having to offset the so-called neurovegetative autonomous functions. This means that what normally functions automatically and subcortically should ideally be restored in the same manner, so energy losses can be avoided. It's a little like putting an end to taking the longer route (from the cortex to the relearning behaviour) and establishing a routine towards neuronal short-cuts (not consciously remembering that it is better to chew when you are eating or that you need to breathe through your nose, but allowing the body to reappropriate its rythmic subcortical functions). A financial analogy can be made here: it is preferable to always use the same current account (unconscious and automatic subcortical functions) to handle monthly and routine expenses instead of dipping here and there into your long-term investments (neocortical) that have other objectives and purposes.

We are now speaking about neurovegetative reeducation, namely, a reorganization at the psycho-neuro-immuno-endocrine level, because psychological means neurological, hormonal and immune system-related, given that everything is related!

To be effective, energy conservation is affected along the way by the recovery of the body's vital rhythms and compliance with environmental rhythms that govern us. These rhythms are deficient in all of us who suffer from an energy deficit (starting with respiratory rhythm). This deficiency results in an imbalance, hence the loss of energy efficiency and the vicious circle that amplifies the internal disruption. This topic will be covered in Chapter 7.

Conserving one's energy capital also means taking into account emotion and its energy effect that we feel when faced with events and our environment. Also involved is the issue of integrating the balance recovery programme in each dimension of human activity, as suggested by the findings provided in Chapter 3, summarized as follows:

- Rebalance the autonomic nervous system (ANS) by stimulating its
  Parasympathetic branch.

- Acknowledge your apprehensions to eventually find the necessary
  Courage towards a better state of being.

- Rediscover the perception of daily
  Pleasure.

- Realize the need to take care of your
  Self first and especially.

- Regain your personal
  Power.

To better remember these approaches myself, I called this habit-changing method the *PCPSP programme*. It will help you to understand how the type of energy investments that you made in the past could lead you to bankruptcy and it will give you ideas on how to consolidate your debt, while suggesting strategies for achieving better long-term investments.

What would be good to remember is that, both financially and energy-wise, one must always pay interest before paying off a debt!

Exercise 1.1: Energy stages

Now that you have quantified the manifestations of your energy exhaustion with the help of Tables 1.2 and 1.3, observe them in relation to Table 1.4 and ask yourself in what energy stage you find yourself today.

Once you have assumed in which stage of energy imbalance you find yourself, use your result from Tables 1.2 and 1.3 and enter the totals of the physical and psychological manifestations in their respective boxes in Table 1.4, based on the stage in which you believe yourself to be. Hold on to your results dearly. You will be able to use them in the future to motivate yourself on days when your energy is lacking, when your morale is down and, consequently, when perception is too subjective and energy-draining to find any comfort. This table is particularly useful to therapists for confronting those individuals who are still in denial regarding the scope of their condition and who, finding themselves in the bankruptcy stage, continue to wear themselves down: the visual aspect helps the person who resists modifying their habits to gain a sense of awareness of the situation.

TABLE 1.4 Energy stages: from imbalance to balance

DATES OF THE SELF-ASSESSMENTS:					
	RESULTS OF SYMPTOMS ACCORDING TO TABLES 1.2 AND 1.3				
Alarm	Physical				
	Psychological				
Recovery	Physical				
	Psychological				
Resistance	Physical				
	Psychological				
Exhaustion	Physical				
	Psychological				
Bankruptcy	Physical				
	Psychological				
Consolidation of debt	Physical				
	Psychological				
Conservation of energy capital and decrease of symptoms	Physical				
	Psychological				
Return to a state of health with less than 25% of the initial symptoms	Physical				
	Psychological				

All the patients who consulted me and who were not feeling their body in the initial assessment with Table 1.2 (with a result between 45 and 55), but who complained of being exhausted, had a result greater than 100 once they became more in touch with their body and this was after only a small number of treatment sessions. These individuals gradually reconnected with bodily sensations that they had banished in order to survive. At this point, it is very important not to conclude that these people's condition is worsening because the physical complaints are increasing. They need to be reassured and understand that their level of awareness has improved and that it is part of the rehabilitation process.

Continue with your detective work. You will certainly discover possible avenues that will explain your current state, at least in part. This data is valuable in terms of being the most objective possible in your work and as a motivator. You are an explorer in uncharted territory. From among the tools available, use those that seem relevant to you. To each his own style, exploration, and choice of tools.

Chapter 2

The Environment in the Twenty-first Century

The more scientists isolate and zoom in on what they study, the less some of them can observe the context as a child would, to thereby understand the global context of what they study.

In Chapter 1 we saw how excessive stress can lead, after many phases of adjustment, to *imbalance and even energy bankruptcy*. When, in order to regain this balance, we want to make changes in our life to better manage stress and, if possible, avoid certain stressors, logic requires us to first identify which factors in our general environment could represent a source of stress. In other words, we want to find the potential factors of serious imbalance in our state of health. To be sure of whether certain elements are stressors that affect us personally or not, we should observe our reactions and our responses in certain contexts.

Observe and question, observe and move forward, observe and grow

Curiosity is a catalyst to making informed changes in our path of life.

Can a virus or a parasite be the physiological cause of this imbalance? Can a lack of biodiversity on our plates be partially responsible for the stress that invades us? Is it sensory and visceral hypersensitivity that makes me more receptive than others – many people don't feel a lot, unless they are bombarded by sensory stimulation – or is it a hormonal, mineral, post-partum vitaminic imbalance, or more than one of these possibilities? Does my body truly speak to me and do everything in its power so I listen to it, making me finally decide to rest?

All questions, even the most unlikely, are valid when you don't know what you are dealing with. Opening yourself up to ancient wisdom can provide you with additional tools. The goal is not to find a specific cause, but rather to fit together several pieces of the puzzle and begin to see a little more clearly what originally affected you and what continues to affect you – which can help you heal without hiding either the symptoms or emotions. When experiencing symptoms, it is essential to understand the mechanisms of stress by taking note of their frequency and of the events that exacerbate these symptoms. Finally, it is important to resume this very observation work when you change your approach. Why observe? To take a step back and put things in perspective, to avoid sinking into a depression or shifting into panic mode, to find liberating solutions (leaving behind the 'why' and adopting the 'how'), and especially, to move forward, learn, and grow.

Observing is not judging, feeling guilty, having regrets, placing blame on a source outside of yourself, wallowing over your lot in life, or getting worked up over useless anxiety when faced with challenges. It's an exercise in patience which is accomplished over time, a work of precision and consistency, carried out with detachment.

Reflecting on our environment: a few facts

A study done in 2007 and 2008 on 232 toxic substances we find in human tissue in newborns and another study show body[1] burden levels of hexachlorobenzene in the general population in the United States. These data prompt us to question our *power to adjust* to these toxic substances that increase from year to year in the environment and, incidentally, within ourselves as well, because we form an integral part of this environment. Pelt and Séralini specify that scientific data exist that demonstrate the relationship between 'chemical molecules and various physiological disturbances that can affect the nervous, reproductive, respiratory, and even immune systems'.[2] Wouldn't one of the most insidious effects of our collective poisoning – that occurs slowly but surely – by way of chemicals, ultrarefined junk food,[3] petrochemicals, certain plastics,[4] legal or illegal drugs, and all types of toxins be to challenge the possibility that we can adjust to the psychosocial stressors of our everyday lives?

It is nevertheless the stressors which are underestimated because they require the same adjustment process as psychosocial stressors.

Chemicals can also 'act in a combined fashion and be transmitted from one generation to another'.[5] In addition, some chemicals potentiate the adverse effect of others.[6] Allergic reactions that have not been or have been poorly identified appear among the other imbalances of the body–mind towards which this insidious poisoning leads us. Over time, this toxicity can be transformed, according to each individual's genetic baggage, into degenerative and auto-immune diseases, even into cancer.[7]

Personal observation

In May 2008, when my health had recovered for more than two years, I was on the job market and was taking a karate class two to four times a week, I had to go to the dentist so he could change two dental amalgams that I had had in my mouth since I was a teenager. Not even an hour had gone by since I left the clinic that most of the symptoms of myalgic encephalomyelitis reappeared along with a sharp pain in my jaw and throughout the entire nervous distribution of the trigeminal nerve. Physically, the diffused pains, the trembling, the sudden energy lows, and the severe functional hypoglycemia came back. Over the next three months, my menstrual cycle shortened and the flow became heavier once again. Emotionally, I once again became short-tempered and impatient and my autonomic nervous system (ANS) was in sympathetic mode most of the time, even when at rest. I had neck pain on the same side as my teeth that had been treated and the lymphatic nodes in my neck and armpit were sensitive and swollen on the same side. On a cognitive level, I started losing my memory, re-entering a state of disorganization. I had to once again start taking supplements to reduce the symptoms. I became open to the possibility of mercury poisoning and I entered a detoxification programme. Despite my initial skepticism, several symptoms disappeared only a few days after I had started the programme. In August 2008 I had to have two other old mercury amalgams changed, complicated by the added procedure of a root canal. This time, I immediately initiated the detox protocol. Several symptoms appeared, but the nightmare was very short-lived and much less intense.[8]

J. G. Lipson draws an analogy between individuals suffering from *multiple environmental sensitivities*, a problem associated with *energy imbalance*, and the canaries that the miners brought with them into the mines to ensure air quality – the volatile canaries were the first to die in the event of gas poisoning...[9] At the other end of the spectrum of this same discourse, Richard Leakey, a paleoanthropologist, and Roger Lewin, a biologist specializing in the ecology of evolution, 'propose that we are currently experiencing the sixth mass extinction of species'.[10]

Patient's observation

Sonia is a cleaning woman who feels good and energetic in the homes of her two clients who use environmentally friendly cleaning products. On the three other days, she coughs, complains of sinusitis, and feels mentally confused when she uses cleaning products that contain phosphates and Javel water. She made a connection between the products used and her breathing problems but she says that unfortunately she cannot change jobs.

Overpopulation–overpollution

> *In the twenty-first century we carry an environmental burden*
> *that taxes the health of each new generation a little more.*

At the beginning of the nineteenth century, the global population was estimated at one billion individuals. In only two hundred years, this number grew by five billion individuals: a first in the history of humanity. It is estimated that, by 50 years from now, this could increase by another five billion.[11] This unprecedented success in the birth rate and the survival rate has had a direct impact on the sustainability of food production methods since the beginning of the twentieth century. These production systems expose our bodies to all kinds of foreign substances (growth hormones, antibiotics, pesticides, herbicides, and chemicals), and deplete what is on our plates and in our water – a true depletion even if, for only a brief moment, we end up feeling satiated.

Note that the deficits in minerals required for the brain to function properly seem to prevail among violent criminals,[12] as compared to the existing deficit among individuals who have committed minor criminal acts. Dr Carolyne Dean specifies that the existing North American diet has a calcium-magnesium ratio that is between 5:1 and 15:1, while that of our ancestors had a Ca-Mg ratio that was richer in magnesium, that is, around 1:1.[13] 'In Canada, the prevalence of asthma has quadrupled over the last decade and 11.2 per cent of Canadian children under 15 years of age suffer from asthma.'[14] It is often linked to an intracellular magnesium deficiency.[15]

Psychiatrist Andrew Stoll drew a connection between the current significant dietary imbalance in Omega-6 and Omega-3 fatty acids and the change in our eating habits, even though this change has only existed for a few generations. We would have gone from an Omega-6 and Omega-3 ratio of 1:1 to 10:1 and even to 20:1.[16] Dr Servan-Schreiber notes that 'a diet deficient in Omega-3 reduces the experience of pleasure!'[17] A change in behaviour in rats lacking Omega-3 is also observed: more anxiety, learning difficulties, and panic experienced in stressful situations.[18] A deficiency of Omega-3 would have an effect on the inflammatory process of people suffering from cardiac disorders, rheumatoid arthritis, mood disorders and, possibly, in children with attention deficit disorders.[19]

Learning deficits are also on the rise in our western society and they are also linked to a deficient diet.[20] Psychiatrist Larry Christensen draws a connection between nutritional deficiencies among volunteers placed in a state of semi-starvation and mood changes.[21] He also noted in some of his patients that the single act of eliminating sugar and coffee from their diet reduced symptoms of anxiety and depression. Is stress something that we would find on our plates? Nevertheless, all of our medical beliefs since the twentieth century have been based on a system whose foundations are completely different and within which there have never been so many specialists available to address our emotional and mental state and so many prescriptions for happiness and sedation pills. So where lies the error?[22]

Our global consumption of fossil energy is also a problem. Even though few scientific organizations rush to conduct valid and reliable studies to prove it on humans, scientists are busy observing the effects of petrochemicals and other chemical substances that act as pseudo- or xeno-hormones and interfere with the hormonal balance of animal species and therefore most probably with ours as well![23]

Our contact with the physical environment

> *Our sense of touch defines the physical boundaries of who we are in relation to our environment.*

The physical environment is in contact with our body–mind through our senses. Our senses act as *translators* of information that the environment communicates to our nervous system. Information is an *energy* that is sent to the body–mind through the senses, which have a direct connection to the primitive brain in which our ANS is located. It is estimated that approximately 80 per cent of our ANS is made up of sensory fibres. The senses therefore have a special bond to ensure our survival in the environment, about which they send us information.

Since the end of the last century, several of our senses have been working overtime. The more the sensory sensors are consistently stimulated, the more they adjust and modify their tolerance threshold. But the nervous system cannot adjust inordinately without giving the brain the necessary time to rest. Auditory hyperstimulation, nights that are no longer dark, and artificial and toxic olfactory emanations increasingly involve our senses. Furthermore, each person is born with a different way of processing sensory information. By basing their work on the initial works of Jean Ayres, several occupational therapists working with children suggest and demonstrate that there exist two major sensory processing patterns of integrating information from our senses: sensory avoidance, due to very high sensory sensitivity, and sensory seeking which, on the contrary, most often results from a weak recording or from weak sensory integration.[24] The first behaviour can be summarized as being the *reflection of a hypersensitivity* and the second one as being a *hyposensitivity*. These two approaches adopted by the nervous system for organizing how sensory information is received influence the way in which we perceive the world. Generally, for each sense found in the human mosaic, there are people who are hyposensitive and others who are hypersensitive. It is therefore possible to be hypersensitive to sound and hyposensitive to deep touch.

This would perhaps partially explain why certain people have a more or less high tolerance threshold to stressors. If you suffer from persistent fatigue, you have surely noticed that one or more of your senses react more sensitively than before. In other words, you have become hypersensitive to sound, odour or light... There is a *sensory overload*,[25] as seen in children with attention deficit disorders and pervasive developmental disorders. In people suffering from persistent fatigue, this often results in sensory avoidance that gradually settles in daily. All these subtle changes suggest a sensory integration difficulty. They would reflect a lack of organization or a neurological imbalance, more or less serious, depending on the situation. It is as if the brain, our mainframe, which is already burdened with too much information to process, was reacting to the smallest piece of newly sent information.

Personal observation

I became aware of the fact that I was unconsciously avoiding breathing through my nose when I was outside, in an urban setting. I took note of this phenomenon when it started, in about 2000. When I was in my worst condition, I noticed a direct impact right away when I breathed close to a truck with a running motor or to a house whose tar roof was being redone: I became irritable, my sympathetic nervous system became upset, I was nauseous, and I would often come down with a migraine in the minutes that followed. My children noticed these reactions, pushed me to close the car windows to block overwhelming odours. Knowing that smell is directly linked to the limbic brain, perhaps these stressors were leading my emotions by the nose at the time...

In Appendix 3, you will find a list of physical stressors influenced by, or exerting power over, the senses. Without knowing if they are affecting you or not, check off what your senses are exposed to on a regular basis. This will give you an idea of the way in which you are using, or possibly *mis*using, your senses.

The social and cultural environment

The belonging group can be considered a *superorganism* in which each individual acts as a 'sensory organ and motor for the whole, contributing to the well-being of the group and drawing upon its collective experience'.[26] This observation also proves to be accurate for energy-draining emotions: if a person in the group becomes anxious, this will have anxiety-provoking consequences on the other members of this group. We know that an environment within which people argue a lot is a stress factor and has a harmful effect on the immune system.[27] Any psychosocial change and any cultural context therefore have an impact on our body–mind.

In Chapter 1 we addressed the influence of psychosocial changes on our PNI system. These changes are better known in medical literature than changes in the physical environment, and consequently will often be factors recognized by the physician or the psychologist, leading them to offer either an adjustment disorder diagnosis or another psychiatric diagnosis.

If you have not already completed the Holmes and Rahe Social Readjustment Rating Scale in Table 1.1,[28] I suggest that you do so now and hold on to your data to use it later on in this chapter. If nothing jumps out at you, do this exercise while thinking of the circumstances in your life six months before the symptoms appeared; the result will be more striking for some of you than for others. In the sixties, Holmes and Rahe developed the Social Adjustment Rating Scale based on this hypothesis. Those researchers included 43 events on which the ratings were based on the degree of adaptation required (see Table 1.1). Even though this list is neither very up-to-date nor exhaustive, it at least provides us with a good starting point for understanding what is going on. The word *change* often reappears as a criterion on this scale. According to the authors, people with a result below 150 feel only minor stress; between 150 and 199, they experience mild stress; between 200 and 299, moderate stress; and over 300, they feel severe stress that leads to serious illness or an accident in 80 per cent of cases. Circle the degree of stress for each event you have encountered in your life over the past six months and calculate the total to discover your psychosocial stress level.

The tolerance threshold

Why are certain energy-draining symptoms on the rise?[29] If we compare the stress level associated with today's lifestyle with that at the start of the century or even with the pace of life only 30 years ago, we realize that the demand for adjustment never stops growing (adjusting to a lifestyle that is always increasingly fast-paced and taxing, adjusting to a deficient diet, adjusting to a rising level of pollution, to constantly changing work demands, barring rest periods in our excessively hectic schedules, etc.). Even children find that the summer goes by too quickly while, from our perspective, at their age, the summer was so long, so peaceful and, often, without the constraints of summer camp or soccer training, swimming, theatre rehearsal schedules…and it was nevertheless so creatively fulfilling. We had the time to do nothing at all…and to dream.

Furthermore, we live in a world that requires us to constantly be aware of danger: we need to be on the lookout for paedophiles, terrorists, the water that we drink, the food that we ingest, poisonous material, unhappy individuals who enter schools armed with rifles, etc. Many of us 'multitasking neocortical westerners' find ourselves abnormally – and continuously – functioning in survival mode! It is difficult to think when all we are doing is reacting and perceiving almost everything with apprehension-tinted glasses.

Before the beginning of last century, it was perhaps neurasthenia that best qualified the symptoms that resemble what we are experiencing today. The impact of historical events (the First and Second World Wars, the Industrial Revolution, the Great Crash, etc.) had an effect on the prevalence of these symptoms. What seems to be taking shape at this turn of the century is a phenomenon whereby more and more people are slipping into a state of *persistent fatigue.*

The tolerance threshold of our adjustability is demonstrated in Figure 2.1. This threshold differs from one person to another, but if we assume that it remains relatively stable for an individual over the course of his adult life, we can then compare this individual's flexibility when stressors start to continuously accumulate in his life. The more demands that are placed on an individual's need to adjust, the more that individual approaches his maximum tolerance threshold: this is what is illustrated in Figures 2.2 and 2.3. Once this threshold has been exceeded, the individual will be in a state of PNI imbalance, that is, he will no longer be able to effectively deal with any type of change. According to Dr Brian Luke Seaward, approximately 80 per cent of diseases are caused by stress…[30]

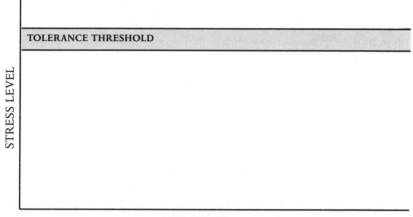

FIGURE 2.1 Basic tolerance threshold to stress

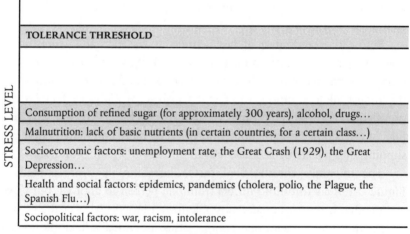

FIGURE 2.2 Tolerance threshold to common stress factors
in a particularly stressful historical context (1930s)

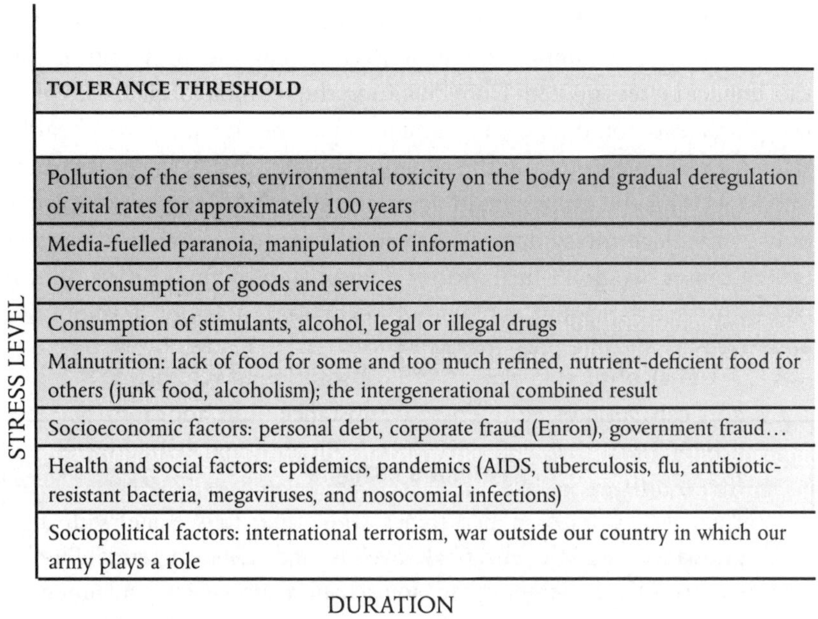

TOLERANCE THRESHOLD
Pollution of the senses, environmental toxicity on the body and gradual deregulation of vital rates for approximately 100 years
Media-fuelled paranoia, manipulation of information
Overconsumption of goods and services
Consumption of stimulants, alcohol, legal or illegal drugs
Malnutrition: lack of food for some and too much refined, nutrient-deficient food for others (junk food, alcoholism); the intergenerational combined result
Socioeconomic factors: personal debt, corporate fraud (Enron), government fraud…
Health and social factors: epidemics, pandemics (AIDS, tuberculosis, flu, antibiotic-resistant bacteria, megaviruses, and nosocomial infections)
Sociopolitical factors: international terrorism, war outside our country in which our army plays a role

(vertical axis label: STRESS LEVEL)

DURATION

FIGURE 2.3 Tolerance threshold to factors
related to the twenty-first century

Evaluation of risk factors

More and more people are suffering from syndromes and diseases that have persistent fatigue as an incapacitating syndrome. That said, we observe that several of these diseases have an immunological component. Can we make the hypothesis based on which this evidence would not depend only on genetic baggage, but also on each individual's environment? Why? Because for at least three generations, our body has been defending itself against the subtle assaults hurled by pollution since it was a foetus, as well as the harmful effects of junk food, refined sugar, and the planet's overall imbalance, combined with the stress caused by daily life, which seems to grow faster and more intense daily.

To make an objective analysis, once you have recounted the striking life events, you need to put these symptoms in perspective, that is, to see the relationships that they support with potential stressors. Whether you consider these stressors to be positive (a wedding or a victory achieved by your hockey club) or negative (an accident, the death of a loved one), they have an impact on your PNI system and it is critical that this impact be recognized. Understanding the multifactorial causes of an *energy imbalance* could have a favourable impact on the return to a healthy state: for example, is it only the situation at work that is the cause of the imbalance or is the cause a multifactorial context? As long as we strive to only camouflage the symptoms instead of focusing as much as possible on the causes, we don't heal. And it doesn't stop there; we then run the risk of further damaging our state of health and, possibly, developing a more serious, degenerative, disease.

Patient's example

Marylin is a woman in her sixties who came to see me with a diagnosis of myalgic encephalomyelitis and joint hypermobility syndrome. After undergoing the biomechanical assessment explaining certain pains caused by the hypermobility of certain joints, Marylin completed my full questionnaire on PNI imbalance: no stressor from her existing physical and psychosocial environment could explain her dramatic physical weariness. When I asked her about her medical history, Marylin finally recalled that she was told that she had had meningitis when only a few months old. During her entire childhood, her father treated her as if she was lazy, incapable, and inactive. She remembers never having had the physical stamina of her brothers and sisters. Following her assessment, I recommended that she adjust some of her habits relating to biomechanics, change her physical exercise programme (because yoga was putting excessive pressure on her joints), consult an osteopath or a physiotherapist for her spinal pain, and continue her cognitive therapy programme centered around mindfulness (based on the principles of Jon Kabat-Zinn[31]) that she had already tried before with a well-known therapist. I suggested that she inquire among health professionals who could help her in terms of energy by pointing out possible after-effects of meningitis on her energy level – as proposed by the theory according to which a virus can be involved. Marylin chose to consult a homeopath. She called me a month later to thank me for having opened her mind and for advising her to take other avenues to restore her health. She has felt better and invigorated since she began following her new programme.

Exercise 2.1: Individual history and stressors

Here is a tool that is useful for you and for the professionals whom you intend to consult in an effort to restore your health. Use Table 2.1 to help you complete your medical history and, at the same time, to highlight the noteworthy facts about your life, on a sociocultural level, relating them to the physical environment in which you have lived. It is important for you to be able to draw your own connections between these events and your medical history. This table will be able to facilitate such a task. However, be wary of hasty conclusions! Be factual. Don't look for problems where they don't exist. Note the coincidences and you will perhaps see a pattern once you have completed the work.

Here are a few examples to help put you in the context:

- Did you feel depressed after suffering from a serious viral infection?

- Have you experienced losses of energy, memory, concentration since you had your car accident, broke your leg, moved into a new house (the house is perhaps contaminated by mould or toxic products stemming from the renovations that you carried out)?

- Is it the fact of being under pressure because of your tardiness, or smog that's making you more irritable when you are stuck in traffic at rush hour?

- Do your allergy symptoms, multiple sclerosis, arthritis, or hypothyroidism tend to worsen with pregnancy, a separation, a betrayal, or after you have swallowed a certain type of food?

At first glance, it is possible that we don't notice the relationship between various factors and our health problems. They are not necessarily the direct cause of our feelings of sickness, but they perhaps stem from a progressive accumulation of stressors.[32] Now go back to your findings in Appendix 3 to make objective observations using the incidents that you have checked off as being potential stressors from your environment.[33]

Refer to these observations and to the Holmes-Rahe Social Readjustment Rating Scale in Table 1.1 to discover a noteworthy event that affects you or perhaps affected you in the past, and see this event, not as a simple coincidence, but as an environment that generates or that amplifies stress. Take the time to do it. It is not a matter of triggering a paranoid thought, but rather of shedding light on what distresses you. Saying that it is psychosomatic or somatopsychic does nothing to help identify all the factors from your environment that have an impact on your suffering.

TABLE 2.1 Individual history and environment

PHASE OF LIFE	YEAR	MEDICAL HISTORY	NOTEWORTHY EVENTS SOCIOCULTURAL STRESSORS	STRESSORS FROM THE PHYSICAL ENVIRONMENT
INFANCY				
CHILDHOOD				

ADOLESCENCE			
YOUNG ADULT			
ADULT			

As far as considering depression and anxiety as purely psychiatric conditions, this prevents, in some cases, a much more complex problem from being identified. Acknowledging an auto-immune disease as being genetic does not mean that you are sentencing yourself to a prognosis or that you are being passive – nor does it mean renouncing the idea of finding solutions to improve your situation and even heal if the disease is detected early enough. Take the time to play detective: it's worth it. Avoid becoming increasingly alarmed as you amass more findings: this doesn't improve the situation at all. Observe without judging.

Patient's daily psychological stressor

Celine, a newly menopausal woman in her fifties, signed up for the PCPSP workshops. She was hoping to find a way of reducing her headaches and restoring her energy so she could re-enter the workforce, because she didn't want to lose her home. Her SRRS result (Table 1.1) was +550!

Exercise 2.2: Medical family history

From what do your loved ones suffer? If you resemble them in terms of genetics and character, as well as in terms of your habits and life choices, it is then possible that you share some of their genetic, environmental, and behavioural weaknesses. You can also put into context the diseases of your parents, grandparents, uncles, and aunts. Observing the type of family personalities that surround you in your family can provide you with certain clues. Make a list. Maybe you will learn something that you never noticed before. Be objective.

To summarize, in this chapter, you have given yourself key instruments for understanding what affects your body–mind in an energy-draining manner. You will gradually give yourself the necessary means to adjust certain habits. These tools will also be used as barometers of the energizing changes that you will introduce into your daily life.

Chapter 3

From Chaos to Energy Balance

*In the patient's rehabilitation process, therapists often observe
a disorganisation or a regression into chaos just prior to a
leap towards a higher neurofunctional reorganization.*

What type of activities do you tend to do on a daily basis? What type
of attitude best characterizes you? Do you resemble the tortoise who
strives to accomplish one single task at a time or do you act like his
adversary, the hare, who undertakes several tasks at once, without
being able to complete them in time? Are you the type of person who
enjoys strolling along, lounging about, who can appreciate a symphony
orchestra in concert, a 300-page book and lose track of all sense of time,
or are you the type who never misses a single moment, who listens to
dynamic music, who never stops moving until the moment, or until the
very second, your head hits the pillow? To relax, what do you prefer:
the calmness of the country or the darkness of those 'Thank goodness
it's Friday' bars? As far as physical activity goes, do you prefer gentle
activities like yoga or a nature walk, or do you choose to take an aerobics
class or a long bike ride, calculating time and speed, while keeping a
specific goal in mind, such as losing weight or enhancing muscle tone or
improving your personal best?

We all have our ways of balancing – or not balancing – our time
between work and pleasure, and our personal, family, and professional
life. It is possible that during a good part of our existence we have been
successful in effectively managing our daily lives. But at a certain point,
certain choices no longer suit us, and others prove to be wiser. We will
see why.

Persistent fatigue is a symptom of imbalance. Our body reflects the
imbalance that overwhelms us in our daily life. Even if we are under the

impression that we don't have control over the stressors that put strain on us, it is possible for us to regain this control before permanent damage affects our body–mind. It is perhaps even possible to defy the statistics and permanently restore this apparently damaged body–mind.

Each one of our activities makes us spend energy in each of the following dimensions: physical, emotional, cognitive, sociocultural, and spiritual. Certain operating modes are more energizing, while others continually disperse our energy. In this chapter, you will have the opportunity to assess your energy gains and losses in the daily activities found within these five dimensions. Similar to performing a financial analysis, you will assess the energy costs of your daily activities and you will realize that you often spend, before replenishing, your energy bank account. You therefore withdraw more than you deposit. The idea is to draft a balance sheet to be able to eventually better plan and manage your energy.

Creating your own Energy Balance Sheet

In this exercise, you will have the opportunity to learn how to evaluate the ways in which you spend and save energy. To do so, you will have to observe your habits through your daily activities. First, list the activities in what you consider to be an energy-draining day (or any day if you are already in 'exhausted mode') based on the following categories:[1]

- Personal hygiene
  - dressing
  - washing (showering, bathing…)
  - eating.
- Productivity
  - domestic tasks (groceries, cleaning, laundry, finances, meal preparation…)
  - care provided to children, parents, friends…
  - remunerated or unremunerated work (school homework, volunteer work).
- Leisure activities (with family, spouse, friends, alone).

To make the task easier for yourself, use the Energy Balance Sheet in Appendix 4 and write down the activities you perform in a typical day using the proposed model. Select four activities and note their duration according to the following categories and sub-categories: *personal hygiene, domestic tasks, work,* and *leisure.* Choose one activity per category and, if possible, add one more activity for the productivity category. Similar to what we encounter in financial analysis, it is important to draw up a list of your habits in terms of gaining and spending capital energy. What is less relevant here is knowing how you spend it, going into the lesser details of each energy 'dollar.' In this chapter, you will only need to select four or five activities to create your Energy Balance Sheet.

In the same way that you would first learn the financial terminology when creating your financial balance sheet, in this context, it is important to become familiar with the concepts related to the energy of the body–mind entity.

Make sure you read the whole chapter before starting this exercise; you will need to identify and classify your behaviour in each of the five dimensions when exploring your energy status. Once familiarized with the new tools, you will be able to better observe yourself, in each of the dimensions, throughout your energy exploration.

Make a copy of Appendix 4 which you can carry with you throughout the day on which you choose to do the exercise. Hold on to it tightly, because once you have completed Appendix 4, you will need to refer back to it for guidance while you embark on adjusting your habits – as it will be relevant in Chapters 8 to 11. Based on your needs, you will be able to redo your Energy Balance Sheet once you have made certain changes to your habits.

When I lead eight-week group workshops, I ask the participants to complete this exercise only for several activities in their daily routine, because it is difficult, in a single day, to do it for all the activities listed, especially for a person suffering from an energy deficiency! What is important is to understand what is *energizing* and what is *energy-draining* for you. Eventually redoing the exercise, after having made changes to your habits, is highly stimulating and reassuring because the positive effects are very visually striking on the chart.

You therefore possess the necessary framework to carry out your *energy financial statements.* Hold on to it tightly. You will need to refer to it as you read this book.

Are you sympathetic or parasympathetic?

Balance: state of stability that prevents one from falling.

The *autonomic nervous system* (ANS) works automatically, on its own, without us being conscious of it. It is divided into two branches: *sympathetic* and *parasympathetic*. Broadly speaking, it can be said that the sympathetic branch is highly solicited when we find ourselves in a fight or flight situation. It's a little analogous to the gas pedal on a vehicle, which makes us consume a lot of energy. Time after time, we hear people say that they have felt a rise of adrenaline when they had to speak in public, or just prior to taking part in an important meeting or before an interview or even when they found themselves in a dangerous or exciting situation, like tackling a ski hill, skydiving, riding a rollercoaster... In Table 3.1, certain effects of the sympathetic branch are more easily recognizable in your own body.

An alarm state can be very stimulating and enjoyable and, for many people trying to adapt to modern life and the technological era, it is often sought after, either consciously or unconsciously. An actor likes to feel a touch of stage fright just prior to going on stage; a businessman will unconsciously ensure that he arrives just on time for his meeting in an effort to optimize his time: this way, he remains sharp. The *sympathetic* system helps us to improve our performance when we are under pressure, but we have to know that it can only do so on a short-term basis.

As the body strives to achieve balance, the parasympathetic branch is also solicited. We can consider it our brake pedal. It substantially offsets, in several functions, the effect of the sympathetic system. This is what you will realize when you compare their effects in Table 3.1.

As we previously described, stress is an important part of our lives. It is unavoidable and healthy. It enables us to react to the unexpected and survive in the face of danger. It also makes us more alert and better able to function in the short term. But like every good thing, it becomes, when it is excessive in quantity and intensity, not only energy-draining, but toxic. When we find ourselves in a situation that I describe as being a 'state of siege', (i.e. when stress bursts forth from all sides), it's the entire ANS that comes to the rescue. Consequently, we function in 'fight or flight' mode. But if we do not take the time to return to a pre-alert stage – like the gazelle who goes back to his daily routine after having escaped the jaws of the lion who was charging him – imbalance will set in. Modern man remains on guard. He has lost his effort-rest-effort-rest cycle.

In response to stress, the endocrine system secretes multiple hormones. From the hypothalamus to the pituitary, and then to the thyroid gland, the adrenal glands and the sexual glands, the body is activated. The endocrine glands step into overproduction mode. How much longer can they continue to work, to produce – to run on the spot like the hamster spinning in its wheel – until reaching the point of exhaustion? Several other glands produce hormones at an alarming rate and subsequently deplete. The master gland, namely, the hypothalamus-pituitary gland, is overexcited and activated to the point of throwing off its secretion cycles. Our tolerance threshold diminishes in the face of any outside stimulus decoded by our senses. However, another response mode is possible. We will see this response in Chapter 7.

Silence is golden. Be calm and quiet, and observe.

Exercise 3.1: Physical Energy Balance Sheet

Go back to Appendix 4. By considering your bodily sensations and using Table 3.1 of the ANS functions as a guide, enter an X in the *Sympathetic* or *Parasympathetic* column of the Energy Balance Sheet each time you experience a *major change* in your ANS during the four activities selected for this exercise. (For example, it can basically be said that doing aerobic activity triggers primarily the sympathetic system while the parasympathetic system is felt more at the end of exercise, when the body–mind tends to achieve a state of balance. If you do yoga and are successful in truly relaxing, perhaps you are shifting into the parasympathetic mode more while the sympathetic mode discretely readjusts). Certain activities strongly stimulate the two systems (such as organizing a family celebration, preparing supper amidst rambunctious children, etc.): divide up the time if you feel the need to do so (for example: 40% sympathetic and 60% parasympathetic).

TABLE 3.1 Certain effects of the two branches
of the autonomous nervous system

SYMPATHETIC MODE	PARASYMPATHETIC MODE
	Tear secretion (without necessarily being linked to an emotion, like during a yawn)
Dry mouth	Increased salivation
Muscle pain, stiffness in the shoulders, neck, forehead and/or jaw	Sensation of relaxation
Inhibited peristalsis (movements of the digestive tract)	Accelerated peristalsis (movement of the digestive tract)
Increased blood pressure (you feel as if your face is getting red)	Relaxation of blood vessels
Increased heart rate (for example, during an athletic activity or during a heated meeting)	Decreased heart rate
Increased breathing rate	Decreased breathing rate

Do not try to change your reaction; just observe it and identify what is happening unconsciously inside your body. Recognition alone of these facts brings a sense of receptiveness to change. Let go of the inner critics. Do not judge your behaviour; it has been useful to you in order to survive in difficult times in the past. Just observe: that's all! In Chapter 12 we will review different ways of easily restoring a balanced ANS based on the energy level, cognitive functions of the moment, physical tolerance, and environmental and economic constraints.

Fear and courage

Courage is often the first step in an energizing direction.

An emotion is an affective reaction translated by a neurovegetative manifestation. In other words, it is an ANS reaction. It is therefore to our benefit to better understand our own emotions and how they make us feel in our bodies. Improving our awareness of what we feel during daily life activities is a direction to follow in order to discover the underlying motivations of our behaviour during any activity. For many people suffering from persistent fatigue, an older, latent emotion can be the source that offsets the balance of the PNI system. Even those emotions that remain unconscious translate directly into a change in the neurovegetative functions, an influence on hormonal secretion, and an inhibiting or activating effect on the antibody production of our immune system.

Fear is an emotion that can lead to behavioural inhibition.[2] It limits us on a personal level. If we want to foster personal growth, it is preferable that we recognize the emotion of *fear* or, rather, the feeling of apprehension or threat. We then transform this emotional state by stepping back from our thoughts. In Chapter 9 we will discuss in greater detail the approaches to adopt.

'Confronting obstacles develops courage and personality.'[3] If we are courageous, it means that we possess a 'willingness to try new things and deal with the changes and challenges of life'.[4] At this level, we can therefore exercise *control* and *options* and dare to move forward. Research has suggested that depression can be averted when people are given the possibility to find meaning in their daily activities. This renews their feeling of optimism and the possibility of believing that they are exercising options and control in their life.[5]

Exercise 3.2: Emotional Energy Balance Sheet

Several emotional states that often camouflage an inner energy-draining environment, including fear, are listed in Table 3.2. The emotional states that indicate that the stage of courage has been attained and that influence our behaviour in a more developed manner, during activities, are also summarized in Table 3.2. Use this list of emotions when, for each activity selected for your Energy Balance Sheet in Appendix 4, you ask yourself which emotion or state of mind you are manifesting within.

TABLE 3.2 Polarity of Emotions[6]

FEAR (ENERGY-DRAINING EMOTIONS)	COURAGE (ENERGIZING EMOTIONS)
Shame, humiliation, indignation	Courage, assertiveness
Guilt, blame, impatience	Neutrality, confidence
Disgust, agitation, obsession	Inner peace
Cruelty	Goodness
Apathy, despair, pessimism	Goodwill, optimism
Desire, envy	Sense of purpose
Anger hatred, bitterness	Unconditional love, respect, inner peace
Pride, disdain, avoidance, indifference	Joy, serenity
Mourning, regret, denial, disappointment, betrayal	Acceptance, forgiveness, fairness
Closed-mindedness	Open-mindedness
Apprehension, fear, anxiety, suspicion, annoyance, frustration	Understanding, reasoning

You may be confident when you are shopping, angry at work, guilty at home (if you are on sick leave for instance), and neutral when doing the laundry. To each his own! Only today's answer is relevant. Tick off *fear* (energy-draining effect) or *courage* (energizing effect) based on Table 3.2. You very well might find more than one emotion during one activity and on both sides of the table; tick off both sides in that case. If you prefer, estimate a percentage; numbers are familiar points of reference that tend to be reassuring for many people in our modern society, in which the initiatives of quantifying and ranking are very important.

Be honest with yourself. It is possible that you are so disconnected from your emotions that you are incapable of recognizing your emotional state. Accept this observation. You just discovered something and that, in itself, is already constructive. The next section, which is more cognitive and factual, will help you to grasp the fact that you are feeling emotions and, eventually, to differentiate between them.

If an emotion is expressed during the exercise, do your best not to avoid it; acknowledge it head on so it surfaces, unless the circumstances are not so conducive. You will go back to it at a later time. Don't forget that we live in a society that conditions us to receive instant gratification and that, as a result, we are not used to experiencing disturbing emotions. The tendency is rather to dull the feeling. Try not to sink into common avoidance patterns: if the experience is too overwhelming, go and seek help from a friend or a health professional.

Once again, don't judge yourself! Be indulgent with yourself. Observe your approach and your way of being. This is the direction to follow. In Chapter 9 you will find the tools needed to tackle the findings uncovered in this exercise.

The perception of duty and pleasure: obligation or enthusiasm?

Happiness is unrepentant pleasure.

Socrates

The perception we have of any activity is very important as it relates to the motivation required to take part in it, to the emotions associated with it (energizing or draining) and to the physical energy needed to achieve it. *Duty* is perceived as something *required* to be done and, in itself, the requirement is perceived as a burden in which there is no room for creativity. We all show more enthusiasm when we have a particular interest in the subject of the duty or when it is perceived as a game rather than an obligation.[7]

We are now going to consider *pleasure* as being a favourable perception related to the exercise of daily activities for which there is an element of interest. Whatever it is, if the productive or leisure activity is going to be recognized as enjoyable, we need to be interested in it, to perceive it as being in line with our creativity. When this activity is a task, an unappealing burden, we stop bubbling with enthusiasm and we lose our vitality. There are people who bubble with pleasure; whatever they undertake, they have a playful attitude, even if the activity is, in itself, dull and routine. However, others become exhausted by forcing themselves to act and by getting bogged down in 'the duty before anything else'. There are other individuals who feel so stifled by their duties that they avoid and sabotage them. They drag their feet until they hit a state of extreme procrastination.

In the framework presented here, what place do you assign pleasure in your daily life? Do you have little or no time for leisure activities? And even if you do have the time, do you generally seem to be gifted at transforming *pleasure* into *duty*? For example, I 'must' go to the gym, 'I have to' finish this work for the boss or the client... However, do you find these routine activities enjoyable, such as doing the dishes for example – because it's useful for the entire family – or driving in traffic – this way, you can sing along with the pop star on the radio – or going to work with an open, willing attitude?

Sometimes there is a very fine line between enthusiasm and obligation. The fact that we feel more stress than usual (of any kind) can transform someone who derives pleasure from working effectively into a workaholic who survives by maintaining a sense of obligation. Passions can become obsessions. When we are under pressure, our perception shakes our mental side and can render it obtuse and limited. That is when old habits return, in the form of reflexes, to stand up to adversity. The primitive brain, which is necessary to our survival, takes over at this point.

When work in itself is repetitive and monotonous, we may tend to perceive it as an obligation with no intrinsic value other than, for example, earning an income. However, nothing prevents us from being creative when we perform these tasks, whether it be in our approach to dealing with others or in our way of dressing, doing our hair (even if we wear a uniform to work!) or in the way in which we decorate our work environment. 'Creativity is each person's personal touch and is not expressed solely through the execution of the task itself, but also through the ways in which the work place and structures are organized.'[8] All these ways of *being* can indicate the difference between having an interest in doing an activity and feeling obligated to do it. For some people, it is often only the way in which things are perceived that lessens or increases the level of stress.

'It's thanks to the imagination that we are able to adapt, innovate, face an unknown...'[9] If we have been force-fed information since childhood in an effort to make us into little docile, productive soldiers, but without the ability to develop our imagination, through play and arts, we will not have learned what it means 'to be oneself' and be more than the reflection of what others expect of us.

When work becomes perceived as play, I am privileged to have broken free from an energy-draining perspective.

Exercise 3.3: Cognitive Energy Balance Sheet

Return to the previously selected activities to follow your balance sheet (Appendix 4) and learn more about your habits. Review each of the activities entered and, in the *Cognitive* section, indicate with an X the angle of perception through which you approach your daily activities. How much room do you have in your daily activities for pleasure and duty respectively? It is possible that some activities are perceived as having both aspects at once, for different reasons: because of the task being carried out, the environment or the context in which the activity is performed or the attitude adopted. Here again, estimate a percentage if you can.

After having completed this exercise, you may realize that at a certain point in your personal development, you associated a *job* (duty) well done with conditional love. In Chapter 9 we will address different ways of approaching daily activities and occupations.

Who comes first: 'myself' or others?

Love your neighbour like thyself.

Leviticus 19:18

In this chapter the psychosocial aspect will not make direct reference to the environment, but rather to a need we feel while in that environment: our need for self-knowledge and self-esteem. From the need for self-knowledge stems the underlying need for acknowledgement and recognition,[10] which is often disregarded and underestimated in the sociocultural environment (especially the work environment) in which we develop. This is what we are going to explore in this section.

The malaise of doing and of having

Is it the perception from others around you that mainly motivates you or does your motivation also come from within yourself? Do you seek *recognition* that never comes? A motivation that comes only from outside can confine us to a life of deceit, quite simply because we want to please others based on their criteria. This recognition comes at a pretty high price, especially if it is not felt at all, or if it is too short lived. Perhaps you tend to excessively indulge in accumulating equity? Is it so you can advertise your success? Are you the type to perform feats or spread your knowledge for a compulsive need to have relentless public recognition? Wouldn't compulsive 'doers' be addicted to success – even if success can be noble in itself? They are trapped in the vicious circle of winning back the sense of reward by striving to conquer yet another challenge, to fill an inner void, as if they were incapable of enjoying the success in the moment. Neuropsychologist Paul Pearsall sees this as *Toxic Success Syndrome.*[11]

Self-esteem: superiority-inferiority complex

Many people suffering from professional burn-out work in the helping field in the broad sense of the word – particularly in the fields of health and education.[12] Since they do not receive recognition from their superiors or from their work colleagues, they fall into a trap in which they seek this recognition from their students, patients or clients. But the very fact of taking care of others to the detriment of their own needs quickly becomes stifling and exhausting. Although the conscious motivation is virtuous in itself, its unconscious perverse effects are often felt long term. The search for self-esteem is at the root of this motivation. Over time, what we enjoy doing for *others* ends up becoming an obligation when we continually deprive ourselves in order to be able to do this activity. It casts a dark shadow over our way of thinking and drains our energy. We shouldn't delude ourselves; it is sometimes with a sense of superiority that we judge others and take care of them. As for those who have learned that *others* must come before *oneself,* they experience a feeling of inferiority which unconsciously underlies this behaviour.

Exercise 3.4: Sociocultural Energy Balance Sheet

Return to your list in Appendix 4 and ask yourself the following questions:

- Is it an activity that pleases me or do I do it to please others?
- Is it an activity that I do to fulfill my own needs or the needs of others?
- Is this an activity adapted to me or is it imposed by my environment?
- In summary, do I do this activity primarily for myself or for others?

Take note of your proclivity for each of these activities by thinking of your needs and those of others. You will probably see a trend stand out on your table between thinking first of oneself and thinking first of others. In Chapter 10 we will explore the results of your trends in greater depth. We will also address ways of restoring the balance between your individual needs and those of others.

Power versus powerlessness

Emotional vitality reduces the incidence of disease
and improves immune system functioning.

In this context, spirituality will be defined as the dimension in which the human being will place himself when he becomes aware of the fact that his 'I', while being different from others, is in harmony with his overall environment. In other words, although this 'I' is unique, it belongs to a greater whole. Therefore, in this context, *powerlessness* is the impression of having an 'I' that would perceive itself as being alone in the universe, where it must be on its guard, resulting in a deep *malaise*, a deep anxiety. The 'fight or flight' response limits our ways of coping with life. The more the individual needs to defend himself and force things and events, the more he needs to exercise an exterior sense of control – trying to control time, for example, from which stems this crazy race against the clock to which he subjects himself and subjects those close to him – and the more he tries to hide a great powerlessness. Consequently, his internal balance gets worked up and becomes unsettled. A manifestation of powerlessness is recognized by the fact that things are always being forced.

If this style of reaction is unsuccessful or insufficient, a new defence system can settle in, that is, an absence of reaction or inertia. If this system continues long term, it is all the more harmful that it renders us passive in the face of events. This survival mechanism is called the *behavioural inhibition system.*[13] Living with this perception is like learning that, whatever we do, negative repercussions coming from the environment will always strike us. We therefore stop fighting, resign ourselves, subject ourselves to fatality in order to survive. Our body–mind also starts to resign itself, meaning that it fills with toxins and stagnates. And illness sets in, following this powerlessness that transforms into learned helplessness.

Power is an inner feeling of well-being: we are certain that our 'I' is part of a whole greater than us. From this certainty is given off a true sense of humility, which grows, in a process of detachment with respect to the illusory image of an isolation that does not exist. When we feel *powerless* and seek *power*, we can acquire it when we are finally ready to accept what we are, at this point in our lives. The difficulties we face 'contribute to a higher degree of spiritual accomplishment'.[14]

To feel united with humanity, certain people join an exclusive group to which they belong without realizing that this identifiable group can essentially isolate them from the rest of the world. They have an illusion of power, which does not last. In these cases, these people tend to follow the rituals, behaviours and beliefs of the group, whatever they are, ignoring their ability to think for themselves and their integrity. As such, they assign to others their power to choose. Feeling powerless – because they are disconnected from the rest of the world – they indulge in activities that fail to respect what they truly are. Whether the group is family, friends, the religious community, an association, a union, or a political party, there is a danger, albeit subtle, because these people avoid standing up for themselves and taking their place, thinking for themselves, in order to make informed choices. They are in fact avoiding using their own power.

To conclude, we can say that the most *powerful* of beliefs is the one in which we feel connected to the rest of the world and in harmony with the universe. We know our place, our purpose, and, as much as possible, we live based on our aspirations, values, goals, that is, our mission, regardless of how humble it is. And the most *powerless* of beliefs is the one in which we feel completely alone, in which we know that we are not part of a whole and that we do not contribute anything to what makes up our microenvironment.

Everything is related.

Buddhism

Exercise 3.5: Spiritual Energy Balance Sheet

For the last time, return to the activities you chose to do for your Energy Balance Sheet in Appendix 4. In order to know if you engage in your four activities with an attitude of power or powerlessness, ask yourself the following questions. They will help you in your work.

Are you forcing yourself (powerless)?

- Do you tend to force things and events?

- Are you efficient, quick to respond, without a smile, a pause, a joke, some degree of silliness?

- In your own mind, are you entitled to make mistakes? Do you feel the people around you are entitled to make mistakes?

- Are you so intense that you tend to forget the little joys of daily life?

- Do you try to control others?

- Do you do an activity without assistance to make sure the work will be done properly?

- Do you make sure your spouse, child, parents, employee or business partner never waste their time and are as efficient as you are?

- Do you harbour a sense of unfairness while do this activity?

- Do you always try to make a better deal, get more for your money, make sure you are using all of your precious time in the day following a full and rigid agenda to complete everything you wanted to do?

- During your free time, do you optimize your travel time? Does moving from one activity to the next somehow become robotized and do you end up losing your spontaneity? Are you anxious to do the activities that you consider insignificant (brushing your teeth, doing laundry, taking a shower, etc.) in order to concentrate on continuously more demanding obligations (work performance and leisure activities)?

Are you resigned and passive (powerless)?

- Do you let other people do the tasks or make decisions in your place in order to avoid being held responsible?

- Do you choose to do an activity that is below your level of competence in order to avoid responsibilities?

- Are you reluctant to make decisions or do you avoid making decisions as much as possible?

- Do you avoid positions of power?

Do you assert yourself (powerful)?

- Are you more the type to allow life to guide you without trying to force things, people, events, while asserting yourself?

- Do you attach an intense importance to small details and to daily *pleasures?*

- Do you do your best with the resources at hand without always trying to do more and push your limits further and further?

- Do you take the time to rest, even if you are considerably late in your work predictions?

- Can you find time for your family despite the responsibilities pressuring you?

- Can you express your needs clearly and calmly and act upon them toward fulfilment?

Whether we are being forceful or *passive*, powerlessness is *energy-draining*. Power is *energizing*. It is up to you to make this observation and to decide how you are going to spend the energy you have.

To guide you, here is an example taken from daily activities:

Driving your car

Are you forcing yourself?

- Are you excessively attentive to what is happening on the road or to what you should do to reach your destination?

- Do you engage in an ongoing emotional or passionate mental conversation with other drivers that you consider incompetent?

- Do you feel compelled to turn on the radio to fill a void or to maximize further things you can do while driving?

- Do you try, at all costs, to save a minute, to run an amber light, and to pass using the slow lane while driving on the motorway?

- Do you use your mobile phone compulsively, as well as the email service on your handheld device, your dictaphone or lipstick, so as not to waste an instant, to convince yourself that you are highly pragmatic?

Are you passive?

- Do you avoid driving in the fast lane on the motorway to in turn avoid having someone drive too close behind, thereby forcing you to accelerate?

- Are you more than courteous, yielding your turn at road junctions to others, while convincing yourself that you are not making a mistake?
- Do you avoid driving as much as possible?

Do you recognize your power?

- Do you appreciate your vehicle while you comfortably travel from one place to another?
- Do you notice the first signs of a change in the seasons, the blue sky, the sun that warms you when you are waiting at a red light?
- Do you sing along with the radio when it is playing?
- Do you smile?
- Are you courteous when you drive?

In Chapter 11 we will see ways in which you can regain your *power*.

Summary

This chapter is an exercise comprised of five phases, which correspond to each of the five dimensions. Now that it is done, you have a better idea of what causes you to lose your energy stock on a daily basis. You have certainly noticed that, for each of the dimensions, the left-hand column is the more *energy-draining*, while the right-hand column is a tool intended to boost your energy stock. You have certainly also noted that certain activities could be transformed into energy rather than into an energy loss, a loss resulting in *persistent fatigue*. This simple observation is one of the key points designed to open your eyes to your energy potential and enable you to make better decisions in how you spend this energy. I wish upon you tenacity, courage, and discipline in this process. This is a huge gift that you are offering to yourself.

Have sufficient compassion so as not to judge yourself on your journey; this will make the task easier. And nothing prevents you from asking for help along the way to motivate you to persevere. The task isn't accomplished overnight. Individuals who are still high performers will have trouble finding time for themselves to complete these exercises, not to mention all the resistance they can exhibit while rationalizing why they should not be doing this type of analysis. Bedridden people will have more time, but could succumb to a sense of numbness and choose to mask their weaknesses and remain powerless because they are perhaps not yet at the stage of having courage. Some others will be unable to do this work on account of excessively severe cognitive losses. They will first require a type of therapy that will have an impact on their parasympathetic rhythms in order to restore a minimum level of concentration to ultimately benefit from this exercise. Not everyone is ready to let go their level of perception and analysis, either because they have had inadequate tools over the course of their development, or because they have had too many secretive or unconscious satisfactions, as human nature is so designed. Find your natural rhythm. Rediscover who you really are.

Chapter 4

Physiological Energy

*Basal metabolism: Minimum amount of energy required
to maintain vital functions in an organism at complete rest.*

In this chapter we will see how we store and use energy on a physiological level. This physiological level is highly relevant if you are in a state of energy bankruptcy (operating at less than 40 per cent based on the Daily Energy Scale in Appendix 5 – we will come back to this at the end of the chapter). You will learn how to assess your energy level on a daily basis in order to stop slipping into debt, to be able to pay off your debt and rebalance your energy 'budget'. Over time you will discover the intensity at which you can engage in physical activity without any recurrence of symptoms, which will help you break the vicious circle of energy indebtedness. You will then be able to fill the open gap of which the result is this fatigue that is explained in large part – and more than one thinks – physiologically. The more effective you are going to be, the more your body will be able to heal by itself, once the interest on the debt is paid.

Observe your body.

Breathing–oxygenation

The body is made up of 75 per cent water and it is estimated that oxygen (O_2) constitutes 90 per cent of the weight of this water.[1] Without oxygen, we are unable to 'burn' energy, hence the importance of being well hydrated and breathing well. Every time we inhale, we absorb oxygen, upon which each of our cells depends. Every time we exhale, we discharge waste into the atmosphere in the form of carbon dioxide. We require 3.5 ml of O_2 per kg of body weight per minute,[2] and this is only for the *minimum expenditure of energy* required to sustain breathing, circulation, peristalsis, muscle tone, body temperature, glandular activity, and other vegetative functions performed by the human body. All of these tasks are instrumental in maintaining the dynamic balance of the body, called *homeostasis*. This way of measuring the energy expenditure is called MET or *metabolic equivalent*. The number of METS is equivalent to the quantity of oxygen required for each kg of our weight to carry out any activity. When we are at rest, we spend 1 MET per minute to maintain homeostasis; this is what is referred to as the *basal metabolism*. This is therefore a reference point from which our energy expenditure can be estimated.

Thanks to the equipment available in athletic facilities, we can now find out what we are spending in METS during our training sessions. In our daily lives, it is almost impossible for us to measure our energy expenditure in each of our activities, but we can refer to Table 4.1 to get an idea of this required energy: we will then discover, measured in METS, how much energy is required to carry out certain daily and unavoidable activities, as well as to perform certain leisure activities.

Breathing follows a precise rate with relation to the *oxygen/carbon dioxide* ratio that is immediately required, that is, with relation to both the energy needed and the waste that we create and discard. The autonomous breathing rate is therefore influenced by the energy that we require on metabolic and physiological levels, based on the activity performed, its duration, the position in which we perform this activity, the mental and emotional states and the context in which we find ourselves, in other words, what we are experiencing here and now. Breathing well essentially means inhaling and exhaling effectively based on all these variables. Inhaling is an active process requiring the harmonious contraction of several muscles, including the diaphragm, which plays a major role. Exhaling is moreover passive in nature, although it can also be forced, for example in certain forms of meditation, in order to increase the exchange between oxygen and carbon dioxide. In Chapter 7 we are going to address the topic of restoring a style of breathing that is efficient, that conserves energy – that is optimal and energizing.

TABLE 4.1 **Estimation of energy expenditure per activity**

CATEGORY	ACTIVITIES[3]	METS
Rest	Sleeping	0.9
Activities of daily life (ADL)	Standing up	1.5 to 2
	Dressing, undressing	2 to 2.3
	Washing hands and face	2
Instrumental activities of daily living (I-ADLS) Light work	Desk work (paying bills…)	1.5 to 2
	Sewing (by hand)	1.5
	Driving a car	2
	Peeling potatoes	2, 5
	Doing laundry and hanging clothes on the clothes line	2.5 to 3.5
	Window washing	3 to 4
	Ironing while standing	3.5
	Walking 2 km/h	2.3
	Walking 3.2 km/h	2.5
	Walking 4 km/h	2.9
	Walking 5.5 km/h	3.6
	Walking 5 km/h	3.3
	Walking 6 km/h	3.9
Light to moderate work	Taking a shower	3.5 to 4.2
Moderate work	Walking 6.5 km/h	4.6
	Walking 7.25 km/h	5.4
	Walking 8 km/h	6.9
	Walking 9 km/h	8.6
	Painting, masonry	4 to 5
	Light carpentry	4 to 5
	Raking leaves	4 to 5
	Climbing stairs (8 steps)	5 to 5.5
	Going down stairs	4.5 to 5.2
Moderate to heavy work	Going up stairs	4 to 8

CATEGORY	ACTIVITIES[3]	METS
Heavy work	Masonry	7 to 8
	Carrying 36 kg (e.g. groceries)	7 to 8
	Shovelling (powder snow)	6 to 10
	Shovelling (wet snow)	8 to 15
	Climbing stairs while carrying 11 kg up 8 steps	10
Productivity	Sitting down, inactive, listening to music, watching television	1
Leisure	Desk work sitting down	1.5
	Playing cards	1.5 to 2
	Bowling, playing pool	2 to 3
	Playing golf (with cart)	2 to 3
Small energy expenditure	Playing piano (or other instrument)	2 to 3
	Cycling (10 km/h)	3 to 4
	Horseshoe pitching	3 to 4
	Volleyball (non-competitive)	3 to 4
	Sailing (small boat)	3 to 4
	Fishing	3 to 4
	Horseback riding (posting to trot)	3 to 4
	Badminton (social doubles)	3 to 4
	Playing an instrument with energy	3 to 4
Productivity LEISURE	Hatha yoga, stretching	4 to 5
	Playing drums	4 to 5
	Cycling (13 km/h)	4 to 5
	Canoeing (6.5 km/h)	4 to 5
	Badminton (single)	4 to 5
Moderate energy expenditure	Tennis (doubles)	4 to 5
	Cycling (16 km/h)	5 to 6
	Swimming (not doing laps)	6 to 7
	Ice skating/rollerblading	6 to 7
	Cycling (17.5 km/h)	6 to 7
	Badminton (competitive)	6 to 7
	Tennis (competitive)	6 to 7
	Light downhill skiing	6 to 7
	Water skiing	6 to 7

Productivity LEISURE	Jogging (8 km/h)	7 to 8
	Cycling (19 km/h)	7 to 8
	Horseback (gallop)	7 to 8
	Vigorous downhill skiing	7 to 8
	Basketball	7 to 8
Heavy energy expenditure	Mountain climbing	7 to 8
	Ice hockey	7 to 8
	Cross country skiing (4 km/h)	7 to 8
	Lap swimming (casual)	8 to 9
	Running (9 km/h)	8 to 9
	Cycling (21 km/h)	8 to 9
	Cross-country skiing (6.5 km/h)	8 to 9
	Squash	8 to 9
	Handball	8 to 9
	Basketball (vigorous)	8 to 9
	Lap swimming (vigorous)	10 & more
	Judo, karate, jujitsu, tae kwando	10 & more
	Squash (competitive)	10 & more
	Handball (competitive)	10 & more
	Mountain climbing	10 & more

In tune with environmental sensitivities

According to epigenetics, our genes are affected by our environment and our behavioural choices…

'Normal' air contains approximately 20 per cent oxygen, but in a large urban centre, its concentration can decrease to 10 per cent,[4] hence the importance, when you are a city-dweller, of leaving the city in order to 'clear' the lungs. It is also important to choose where and when you exercise in a city.

If you feel you are affected by environmental pollution, your nose may have been speaking to you for some time already, but you haven't been listening to its messages. Smell shares a direct link with the limbic brain, also called the *emotional and learning brain*. Olfactory memory would have such a powerful impact on the ANS that certain smells could be instrumental in causing a post-traumatic stress reaction: in the case of a soldier, for example, simply smelling an odour related to a memory of the battlefield, such as gunpowder, can be enough to trigger a disproportionate and ill-placed stress response.

With respect to environmental sensitivities, several physicians whose practice encompasses clinical ecology observe that these sensitivities manifest themselves in the form of habits.[5] Initially, there would be a sort of attachment to certain smells to which you have been very often exposed – perfumes, coffee, solvents, gas, turpentine, nicotine, etc. – an attachment that keeps you in a state of dependency (the absence of these smells triggers the appearance of withdrawal symptoms). With time, however, these same smells become aggravating, exasperate us, affect our mood and, in the end, make us sick. Many ex-smokers are good examples of this phenomenon. They are often more intolerant than others toward smokers: without knowing why, they react strongly to smoke. The smell bothers them so much that it triggers a seemingly exaggerated frustration.

Environmental sensitivites to endocrine disruptors

Environmental sensitivities have always been a part of my life. From when I was a teenager, cigarette smoke made me nauseous and gave me headaches. Once I was an adult, perfumes made me sneeze. Tar would trigger migraines within half an hour after having been exposed. The smell of printing ink, bus and truck exhaust gas would alter my mood and detergents would make me nauseous and affect my concentration. During the time in which my energy level was at its lowest (and therefore more and more prepared, that is, in *fight or flight* mode) I was instantaneously bothered by the smells to which I was sensitive: I lost my concentration when I was driving in traffic, or behind a truck emitting foul-smelling exhaust fumes; I felt very tired less than ten minutes after having been exposed to cleaning products… And the worst was that I wasn't sure if all of this was just a figment of my imagination…until I understood that when you have trouble maintaining bodily homeostasis, it takes nothing to throw you off balance!

Careful! Not all exhausted people necessarily develop environmental sensitivities. Every person has genetic and environmental baggage that is specific to him and that makes him more or less vulnerable from an immunological perspective. But it's possible that immunological hypervigilance in certain individuals is one of the causes driving them to a state of energy exhaustion. More and more researchers and physicians working in the field of ecological or environmental medicine observe that exposure to chemical products is a factor contributing to certain types of syndromes with *persistent fatigue* as an incapacitating symptom.[6]

Another sensitive person to endocrine disruptors

I was working with Sophie in early 2002. She was a secretary. After the birth of her child, she developed multiple allergies. She even suffered an anaphylactic shock caused by products used to clean her work space. To reduce Sophie's risk of reaction, the building's cleaning service had to change the cleaning products used on the floor on which she was working.

In Appendix 3 you will find a list of several substances from the physical environment that are stressors which you have perhaps already been affected by, or to which you are possibly intolerant or even allergic.[7]

The Krebs cycle

Nerve cells have an imperative need for glucose. They require about twice as much energy as any other cells in our body.

The Krebs cycle is the chain of cellular chemical reactions that gives our body the energy it needs. Each cell produces chemical reactions within its energy-manufacturing plant. These cellular plants are called *mitochondria*.

We imagine a watermill that turns around and around, transmitting water from one vane to another. The wheel cannot really store energy, but it causes the energy potential to constantly move. This is what is generated within the Krebs cycle. Just as the constantly moving water in the mill transfers energy from one level to the next, there is a chemical reaction that passes energy from one level of the Krebs 'mill' to the next. Adenosine triphosphate (commonly known as ATP) is, within a cell, the molecule that transfers energy, in the form of ions, from one molecule to another, thanks to chemical reactions. The Krebs mill's ability to produce work depends on its ability to extract and use potential energy. In our mill analogy, potential energy is dependent on a waterfall. In terms of intracellular operations, potential energy, which is chemical, is bound to the organic molecular structure. If ATP is to be created within the plant, it needs to be fuelled by oxygen and hydrogen ions. As we have previously seen, we first acquire oxygen through breathing. It is then picked up by the vascular and interstitial channels that send it to each of our cells.

Most ATP molecules are formed by a process that first starts off with food consumption. In decreasing order of energy-production efficiency, we find carbohydrates (sugar), lipids (fat), and proteins – proteins participating at approximately 75 per cent in the synthesis of other proteins rather than in the formation of energy. These chemical reactions process food and retain hydrogen molecules that will be used to form our ATP. It is said that it is an oxidative process, meaning that it requires oxygen (like the oxidization involved in rusting metal). The flow rate of the transportation of electrons, called the *cellular respiratory rate*, is measured as a function of the flow rate of oxygen consumed. We can say that the Krebs cycle is equivalent to cellular breath, the breath that gives us our vital energy.

The entire chemical process of forming and distributing energy in the cellular plants is part of a cycle of complex chemical reactions requiring numerous substances and vitamins or derivatives of vitamins in order to operate properly. In the same way that the wheel of a mill needs each of its bearings to optimally transport its energy, if it lacks an enzyme to help in the production of one or more chemical reactions in the Krebs mitochondrial mill, energy efficiency will be lost, which will exert pressure on the system's internal environment. The operations performed by this Krebs wheel largely depend on the vitamin B complex (B1, B2, B3…) and on magnesium, whose absorption depends on vitamin B6. It's good to note that in a stressful situation, we spend more energy and therefore need more nutrients to feed our cellular energy plants, hence the importance of optimal nutrition.

Muscular energy

We have just seen that energy is produced from what we eat, mainly carbohydrates and fat. The energy used by the muscles is obtained by oxidation of this food, that is, by the chemical reaction with the oxygen available for the muscles. This is called the *aerobic* phase. The oxygen we need for this process comes from arterial blood. The skeletal muscles are unique in that they are able to work during short periods at a level that exceeds the supply of oxygen, which the cardiac muscle cannot do. When the environment is ideally balanced in supply and demand of oxygen, carbon dioxide and water are produced as 'waste'.

If this process is produced in a state in which oxygen is lacking, it is called the *anaerobic* phase. This is what produces lactic acid as 'waste' in our muscles and what stiffens them. It's almost tantamount to the flow of water from the mill being restricted, as if the wheel was turning more slowly and as if the mill was being forced to grind at the same speed. Efficiency declines, overheating occurs (free radicals are produced), resulting in the mill eventually being shut down.

The extreme performance of Olympic athletes, which causes their muscle pains at the end of a race, is a good example of this overheating. The anaerobic phase, which occurs in the absence of oxygen molecules, can only take place when the fuel is glucose. Lipids, which require oxygen to form ATP, cannot bring 'water' to the mill when the incoming oxygen is insufficient. In other words, when you engage in extreme physical exercise you do not burn your pudgy love handles, however, you are lowering your glucose rate. Under these same conditions, if you become hypoglycaemic, in addition to lacking oxygen, you will lack glucose. This explains the energy derailment in many people who suffer from persistent fatigue.

In the case of incapacitating persistent fatigue, it is therefore essential that the one suffering does not engage in intense athletic activity because they lose their energy too quickly and proportionally produce more waste. The symptoms of hypoglycaemia quickly arise in this context of severe imbalance.

Cerebral energy

In order to maintain its integrity, no system can be totally open or closed.

The brain consumes energy in the same way. Despite its relatively small size, proportionally speaking, it is the body's biggest consumer of carbohydrates, hence its hypersensitivity when faced with an inadequate supply of glucose. If your body has been feeling noticeably tired for a long time, there is a strong chance that your brain was sending you subtle cognitive symptoms well before the manifestation of the lack of physical energy that is now preventing you from normally fulfilling your duties.

To summarize, it can be said that energy is generated in our cells from these two vital materials, namely, oxygen and food, and that it is necessary, for our cellular energy mill to run properly, to breathe properly and to consume food that will produce hydrogen ions from *carbohydrates* and *fat*, then from *proteins* transformed into *carbohydrates*. To facilitate and support this incredible transformation and to ensure that our cellular mills are optimally turning, we have specific requirements for certain essential molecules that are commonly part of good nutrition.

An exhausted person is like a high-level athlete. This person demands of his body–mind a very high energy return to pay off his debt and restore his PNI balance.

Daily assessment

In order to continue your detective work observing and trying to establish connections between your state of health and the stressors that have managed to accumulate over the course of your life – I now suggest that you play the role of detective on a daily basis. Perform the following exercise by choosing the scale that is appropriate for you. This exercise will help you to reflect on your cellular energy demand. To assess the daily energy demand required by every individual, I use three scales: the Daily Energy Scale (DES), the Cognitive Scale and the Psychomotor Agitation Scale (Appendices 5, 6 and 7 respectively).

I created the DES over the course of my own rehabilitation, and put the finishing touches to it while treating patients suffering from various conditions and who had persistent fatigue as a common denominator. This scale is useful for people on work disability or who have been forced to limit their daily activities on account of incapacitating fatigue.

As you will notice, this scale proposes, as the first criterion in estimating the body–mind's energy level, to account for the individual's hours of wakefulness during his day, taking into account his need for naps and rest periods. As the second criterion, the scale gives weight to abnormal symptoms of pain and fatigue (see the definitions in Appendix 5). Finally, it takes into consideration the energy level[8] deployed during certain activities in daily life compared to our needs for maintaining the body's homeostasis at rest. To assess the maximum physiological energy demand associated with an activity, I based my assumptions, to assign a numerical value, on certain daily activities whose metabolic rates I was familiar with. In Table 4.1 they are listed based on the energy demand level: light activities < 4 METS, moderate < 7 METS, vigorous > = 7 METS.

When there is a PNI imbalance, the brain's cells – neurons – have the same difficulties as do the muscular cells at maintaining the energy balance – perhaps they even have more, because they proportionally use more glucose than the muscles. To guide me in the choice of the type of activities that was an option for me when I was suffering from a cognitive deficit, I developed a Cognitive Scale. This scale is relevant for people in a state of energy bankruptcy or who are close to such a state and whose concentration has not adequately returned for the DES to be used. If you find yourself in such a situation, immediately go to Exercise 4.2 and use the Cognitive Scale to estimate your existing cognitive abilities.

Finally, the last scale that I prepared targets those who are still 'able to perform' at work or in all of their daily tasks, but who recognize that they are having trouble. I called it the Psychomotor Agitation Scale. I hope it will serve the purpose of an alarm signal for those whose deficits are very close to becoming persistent – which is that much more incapacitating at this operating level.

Exercise 4.1: Daily Energy Scale

If you have less energy than you did before or you feel you are in a phase of resistance, exhaustion, or bankruptcy (as described in Chapter 1), use the DES. Enter what you estimate your energy level to be (as a numerical value or as a percentage[9] as indicated in the DES table). Use a choice of calendar, agenda, or a 'blank graph' on which you can enter the estimate of your energy level for each day of the month. It is important to estimate your score at the end of the day, just before you go to bed or when you wake up the following day to ensure you achieve an accurate approximation for your daily waking hours.

Steps:

1. First, calculate your *active hours* as your first criterion.

2. Consider your need for a nap or a significant rest period.

3. Then take into account the two major symptoms: abnormal pain and fatigue.

4. As needed, monitor your energy expenditure level in METS for a minimum of ten consecutive minutes during your daily activities.

If you decide to use this tool, familiarize yourself with the instrument and make sure to evaluate yourself on a daily basis at the end of the day, before going to sleep, for at least a month. Try to observe and take note of the stressors and the dates on which you make changes to your habits. You can observe, on a monthly basis, the daily fluctuation of your energy expenditures. It is encouraging for some to empirically measure the influences of stressors in one's daily life on their energy level, and the progress that is made on this same energy level, once certain changes have been implemented. I was able to detect, in all the people that I treated, that the road back to health is not linear and works in stages.

At the end of the month, use the chart in Appendix 8a to enter your results. Enter the dates of the month along the x-axis and, along the y-axis, your numerical value between -18 and +5 or the corresponding percentage (in the DES table).

For this scale from -18 to +5, I chose to give 0 as a reference point for the energy level at which we no longer pay interest on the debt when we pay attention to our limitations. Below 0, we always pay interest: the fragility when it comes to maintaining homeostasis is therefore very high. At 0, where we find ourselves at a functional level, we can have a better quality of life while rebuilding the interior of our body–mind and while being capable of maintaining the body's homeostasis. We can withstand certain types of physical stress (e.g. taking a hot bath or engaging in moderate physical exercise of 6–7 METS for 20 minutes) or mental stress (e.g. carrying out intense mental work, feeling strong emotion) without allowing the energy level to collapse. Above 0, we take up a pace completely ahead of that which was driven by an energy imbalance, with a hormonal rebalancing (women's menstrual cycles become more regular and PMS symptoms calm down and then disappear, soft erections in men gradually improve and sudden drops in energy that took place during set periods of the day disappear).

Exercise 4.2: Cognitive Scale or Psychomotor Agitation Scale

If you are in an exhaustion or energy bankruptcy phase, use the Cognitive Scale, as suggested in Appendix 6. In the x-axis of Appendix 8b, enter the dates of the month and along the y-axis, a scale of -10 to 0.

If you have not reached bankruptcy and you believe you are in an alarm, recovery or resistance phase (as described in Chapter 1), you will probably not fully feel the same symptoms as those outlined in the Cognitive Scale. You then correspond to the *tired but wired* type. I therefore suggest that you refer to the Psychomotor Agitation Scale in Appendix 7, which, although less detailed, can help you to figure out where you stand. In the chart in Appendix 8c, you will find along the x-axis the dates of the month and, along the y-axis, a scale between 0 and 4.

Note that the values of this last scale are above normal because they refer to states of hyperactivity – a little as if you were taking a stimulating drug – while what is felt at the stage of the Cognitive Scale is more similar to a craving for this drug. In my opinion, I describe the cognitive slowness as a result of a *marinated* brain (known as 'brain-fag') in which every cognitive function becomes increasingly arduous and energy-draining.

Restoring the wheel of the cellular energy mill

From a physiological perspective, it is clear that better breathing and better eating are two unavoidable factors in restoring our health when we find ourselves caught in the vicious cycle of persistent fatigue. Another condition for success, which is equally important, is to spend less energy, especially the type of energy that makes us even more impaired.

The first thing to do is to make sure you have enough energy for the basal metabolism, especially when functioning below 40 per cent according to the DES (-7 on the digital scale). To maintain homeostasis, you must then choose activities that demand little energy. When you engage in vigorous exercise, since the energy demand is greater, more waste is generated. If your ability to produce energy is impaired, you will tire of producing energy and, to do so, you will have to generate even more toxic waste which, in turn, will demand more energy from you to be eliminated: and the wheel of the Krebs cycle springs even more! Don't forget that a little help is needed to evacuate the toxins that have been accumulating: there's nothing like stretches and manageable physical activity without recurring symptoms to help prevent stagnation in the body.

This way of understanding the lack of energy was never taught to me in university. However, it seems so logical for my clients suffering from a daily lack of energy. This makes sense to them, and in turn makes them feel better. Once they have understood the mechanisms and the symptoms, they learn to control their energy expenditures and investments.

Tips on knowing whether you are maintaining your body's homeostasis

Below 40 per cent (-7) of your energy capacity, you will feel a loss of energy for any activity that causes you to lose your bodily fluids. Battling the summer heat, air conditioning, the deep winter chill, or all three disproportionately exhaust you. Under the same circumstances, you need to dress accordingly and avoid going out, when possible.

Between 40 and 60 per cent (-7 and -3) of your capacity you can do light stretching exercises lying down and short walks outside. But it can happen that you lose energy all of a sudden, hence the importance of planning where, when, and how you spend this energy. Sudden excitement, positive or negative, can easily be a source of exhaustion. Avoid watching the news on television – it tends not to be cheerful – and violent or negative programmes; they weaken your immune system and burn the little that you have managed to rebuild. Remember that it doesn't occur in your head, but actually in your entire body–mind. When you have paid off your debt even further, you will be able to return to this type of environment if you so desire without experiencing a drop in energy.

Impact of exercise intensity on symptoms of PNI imbalance

Three times, my doctor and I realized that I needed to take my return to work more slowly. I started with two half-days for an expected duration of one month. This month was extended by an additional five weeks because my pain, fatigue, and cognitive problems ended up reoccurring. At this point I added two additional half-days for a month, which stretched into two and a half months. It wasn't the motivation that was lacking, but my body had to continue to pay off its energy debt, otherwise it would have continued to mortgage my PNI system.

When you climb back up between 60 and 100 per cent (-3 and +5), you will know that fatigue, intestinal acidity, and pains of an abnormal muscle, joint, or other structure – according to your genetic makeup – are your guides; they warn you when you have done too much. It is difficult to know where the limit is because it changes based on life cycles (seasonal and especially monthly for women), your nutrition, the demands imposed by daily life, and your emotional state. To observe the effects of your level of activity on your body as you become increasingly active, continue to rate yourself based on at least one scale for a little longer. Ideally you would stop the activity carried out before experiencing abnormal muscular and joint pain, cognitive problems, sudden fatigue, and muscular tension. It is important to move, even if it means just stretching on a daily basis, to help eliminate toxins and to maintain one's range of motion in the joints. The less one moves, the more one stagnates and the more one perpetuates the vicious circle of imbalance.

When you obtain between 70 and 100 per cent (-1 and +5) for two to three weeks, you are ready to progressively return to work. It is important to return to work as soon as possible, once you feel ready. Staying at home and constantly delaying this return will cause you to lose energy, and will create a vicious circle of anxiety and excessive anticipation. However, rest assured that this return is done based on your ability to recover because, below 75 per cent, you still have an energy debt to pay.

Making the link between certain activities and lack of energy 1

When Louise came to see me, she had just received a diagnosis of fibromyalgia. She had known for a long time that exposure to perfumes and to the smell of tar, as well as the consumption of chocolate, were giving her migraines. But she needed to use the daily energy scale for three months to take note and recognize the fact that her moderate exercise sessions were giving her a migraine two days after and were increasing her joint pains three days after each session. Louise lowered the intensity and the duration of the exercises, which significantly reduced her pain and the frequency of her migraines. She was able to return to her work gradually and better manage her physical activities and her tendency to push herself too hard.

Making the link between certain activities and lack of energy 2

Carole has been taking care of her handicapped spouse for several years. Her husband's condition has been gradually deteriorating, and she is the only one caring for him daily. She signed up for my workshops and used the DES for six weeks. Through this exercise, she observed that her energy plummeted on Monday and Tuesday of every week. After several weeks, Carole faced the facts: being alone with her husband over the weekend exhausted her while, during the week, since her husband was busy engaging in several activities outside of the house, she was able to go out and relax. This observation led her to understand that she was entitled to ask for help from the CLSC[10] to give her husband a bath and to provide him with the types of care that exhausted her. Her feelings of guilt in relation to this request, that she had never dared to make in the past, faded.

Now that you have an overview of your energy needs at a cellular level, you can explore the ways of choosing and controlling your food sources to regenerate your fuel-depleted body–mind.

Chapter 5

Does Stress Come from Our Plates?

Let thy food be thy medicine...

Hippocrates

Diet and stress

As we saw in Chapter 4, the food we consume is directly related to the energy we can spend. The food that we ingest during the day increases or decreases our vital energy, based on our choices and our consumption patterns.

If we consume harmful, allergenic products, devoid of nutrients, we are asking our body to uselessly spend energy to rid itself of these substances. If we consume too much, we are creating stress and are forcing our body to manage too much waste.

Diet and energy intake

When we suffer from energy problems, it is crucial to have enough vitamins, protein, essential fats, minerals, and carbohydrates each day to use this energy to maintain our metabolism and continue to produce hormones, but also to repair the affected organs. Let's not forget that we pay interest before debt and the creditors prior to making investments! Table 5.1 presents a list of energizing foods and a list of energy-draining foods, which will help you make smarter nutritional choices. Knowing that the Western diet is highly acidating (often because of the quantity of sugar that we ingest), in such a context we can take for granted that a diet that tends to be alkaline in nature is energizing, while a diet comprising more acidating foods tends to be energy-draining.[1]

TABLE 5.1 Food choices: foods that heal and foods that drain[2]

ENERGIZING FOODS	ENERGY-DRAINING FOODS
PROTEIN SOURCE	
Wild salmon Organic poultry Legumes Tofu Organic red meat Organic eggs Nuts preserved in the refrigerator	Any food treated with antibiotics, hormones, herbicides and pesticides Liver (not from organic source) Too much meat = too much Omega-6
CEREALS	
Whole cereals if not intolerant: Quinoa Millet Brown rice Kamut Spelt Rye Oat Wheat Wild rice (not a real cereal, full of protein)	Refined cereals: Commercial cereals Foods made from refined cereals: bread, muffins, pancakes, crackers, sauces, etc. Most likely to be allergenic foods: wheat, gluten, etc.
MILK PRODUCTS	
Organic goat milk Organic cow milk Goat's milk yogurt Kefir Goat butter	All products causing intolerance and allergies including modified milk products, old and soft ripened cheeses Some margarines
STIMULANTS	
	Coffee, tea Chocolate, guaranine Soft drinks
FATS	
Omega-3 and other good fats: Fish and krill oil Flax oil Hemp oil Sesame seeds and butter Other nuts and seeds	Trans fats: Shortening (hydrogenated oil) Fried food Some margarines Most commercial salad dressings Most commercial peanut butter

Salad and cooking oil (in moderation):	Other oils to avoid:
Olive oil Grape seed oil Sunflower oil Safflower oil Canola oil (non-genetically modified)	Cotton seed oil Canola oil
SWEETENERS	
Maple syrup Honey Stevia Strap molasses Dates (without sulphites) Sucanat Xylitol	Refined sugar: fructose, especially from corn source Glucose Aspartame (contains wood alcohol!) Alcoholic beverages Saccharine Cyclamic acid
FRUITS AND VEGETABLES	
Raw vegetable Blanched vegetables Frozen vegetables Fresh fruits Frozen fruits (All preferably organic and/or washed and brushed where appropriate)	All products containing insecticides and herbicides in large quantities (strawberries, cabbage family, etc.)
ADDITIVES	
	BHT (butylhydroxytoluene) BHA (butylhydroxyanisol) Sucroglycerides Food colouring: red, blue, yellow, green (usually petroleum by-products) Nitrites and nitrates Sulphite Monosodium glutamate (MSG)
GENERAL CONSIDERATIONS	
Fresh nuts and oils kept in the refrigerator are energizing Aim to achieve an Omega-6/Omega-3 ratio of 1:1 Our ancestors had a calcium/magnesium ratio of 1:1	Any rancid food Any burnt food Alcohol (can also hide an allergy or intolerance such as wheat, corn, barley, etc.) Current Omega-6/Omega-3 ratio in North American diet -10:1 to 20:1. Current calcium/magnesium ratio in North American diet is from 5:1 to 15:1

The ideal situation would be to have a healthy, balanced diet and eat based on the needs of the body, not emotions, at regular intervals if possible, and in a calm environment conducive to the functions of the parasympathetic system. If you have cravings, find out what your body is trying to tell you. A strong craving for chocolate may suggest you need magnesium. A desire for starchy foods or sugar may indicate a lack of carbohydrates at the cellular level (meaning an intracellular hypoglycaemia) and not a lack of refined sugar in the stomach. If this desire is accompanied by a craving for yeast-based bread or for a fermented product like alcohol, the possibility of *candidiasis* could also be considered: bacteria feeds off these elements![3] A strong desire for alcohol can also mean that you are craving an allergenic product (gluten and/ or corn), or sugar, or any other object of addiction you unconsciously need to calm the symptoms of addiction that manifest themselves in just as unconscious a manner. A strong interest in red meat or liver possibly indicates an iron deficiency. Or a strong desire for salt is in fact a need for iodine – contained in the table salt that we consume in the Western world – which is required to enable the thyroid gland to function; this craving for salt can also be the result of depleted adrenal glands, which cause us to lose certain minerals, a situation that requires a greater intake of trace minerals. It can once again be a deficiency of authentic sea salt, which is rich in trace minerals (table salt and most sea salts have been refined and thereby depleted of 60 trace minerals!). Observe your body. It has its own way of speaking to you.

Food craving can reflect a physical imbalance

Jerome, an obese man in his forties, came to see me with a mixed diagnosis of depression and generalized anxiety disorder. He explained to me that several years ago, his craving for crisps and salt was so great that he would eat an entire large-size bag of crisps when he came home from work…

The less energy you have, the more careful you need to be when choosing what to ingest, however, don't take Table 5.1 as dogma. Use it with judgment. If you have enough energy to 'cheat', do so outside the home, at the restaurant or at the home of friends. This way, you will avoid drawing attention to your problems more than is necessary. On occasion, take pleasure in a little cheating, not with a guilty feeling. If you eat better, you will become less reactive and will be able to handle violating the rule 10 per cent of the time: it's at least two meals a week. Unfortunately, if you have less than 40 per cent of your energy potential on the Daily Energy Scale (Appendix 5), you will increase your debt. It's up to you to judge what is worth the effort. But don't make it into a partisan rule; no one needs a fanatic!

Salt craving and adrenal insufficiency

Several months before I was completely knocked out, my cravings coincided when I finished my karate class (a major energy expenditure) or had a particularly stressful event at work. Afterwards, the salt cravings arose because my adrenal glands were deficient, manifesting in a drop in my blood pressure and very frequent urges to urinate, day and night.

The intakes that you find daily on your plate vary based on your energy needs. If you suffer from irritable bowel syndrome, you could very well require more food than the quantity that constitutes your normal intake, especially if you frequently have diarrhoea. If you suffer from food rather than respiratory intolerances, avoid the foods to which you are intolerant; this will help you enormously! (see the *Food intolerances and allergies* section).

The Western diet generally contains too much meat and not enough fish; the Omega-6 fats derived from meat are excessive in our diet and contribute to the inflammatory process. Try to increase your protein intake by eating fish, like wild salmon and sardines, which constitute an excellent source of Omega-3 (a good fat that the body is unable to produce on its own), and cut down on the quantity of meat you consume. The consumption of red meat is, moreover, an acidifying factor for the body, while we seek more alkaline conditions – which will occur as a result of greater consumption of vegetables and certain fruits with respect to the meat ingested at mealtime.

Digestion and absorption

Things sweet to taste prove in digestion sour.

William Shakespeare

The organs of your digestive system need to be in harmony with one another in order to be able to absorb all the nutritious ingredients of your meals and snacks. Digestion is the process in which food is broken down into smaller pieces, with the help of enzymes produced by glandular secretion along your digestive tract and by friendly bacteria that live in this environment. *Absorption* is the processing of transportation of these smaller particles of nutrients from the digestive tract into the blood circulation. It is the only way to cross the membrane 'check points' and access the digestive blood circulation.

PREPARATORY PHASE (CONSCIOUS, VOLUNTARY AND UNCONSCIOUS, AUTOMATIC)
Ideally, everything begins with the senses! If you cook a homemade meal that emits a strong aroma during preparation, you are in an optimal situation. You are seeing, touching, and feeling what you are preparing, and you are hearing the noise of the utensils, of the water boiling, and of the pans clanging; everything is setting the stage for consumption of the meal. Your salivary glands already secrete a part of what you need to prepare your mouth for the initial stage of digestion. The simple thought of a good meal prepares you for its digestion.

ORAL PHASE (CONSCIOUS AND VOLUNTARY)
Once in the mouth, the teeth chew and grind the food into small portions. The enzymes already begin to digest starches. The lingual lipase is released during chewing. The mucous membranes lubricate the food to transform it into the food bolus for the next phase. If you watch television while you eat, speak on the phone, or if you rush to feed the children and cater to their needs, you are sending less information to your body to adequately prepare the food bolus in your mouth.

PHARYNGEAL PHASE (CONSCIOUS AND AUTOMATIC)
The tongue controls the food bolus and pushes it back to the pharynx. This is how the food bolus goes down the pharynx. The windpipe

briefly closes the airways to allow this passage to the oesophagus to avoid food being aspirated into the respiratory routes. If you are tense and find yourself panting, you will tend to swallow food without having sufficiently ground it, thereby preventing bigger pieces from being properly digested, which will demand more energy from your system for digestion.

OESOPHAGIAN PHASE (UNCONSCIOUS AND AUTOMATIC)
In order for your food bolus to require the least amount of energy possible and sufficiently descend from the pharynx to the oesophagus and then to the stomach, it is important to know that good digestion requires gravity. This implies that it is important to have good posture in a seated position.

GASTRIC PHASE (UNCONSCIOUS AND INVOLUNTARY)
At this level, not a lot of absorption occurs, however, the food bolus is reduced into smaller particles. The ANS parasympathetic pathways are greatly responsible for the proper functioning of this digestive phase, hence the importance of staying calm during digestion. Big, explosive conversations should be avoided. The acid environment of the stomach also helps to destroy undesirable bacteria.

INTESTINAL PHASE (UNCONSCIOUS AND INVOLUNTARY)
The majority of digestion and absorption take place in the small intestine. To digest fat, the intestine must provide alkaline conditions, as opposed to the stomach, which secretes hydrochloric acid. The pancreas and the gallbladder secrete bicarbonate, which contributes to alkalinizing the environment. The liver, which eliminates toxins from the body in bile salts, empties them from its warehouse (the gallbladder) into the intestine. If the contraction (by the parasympathetic nervous system) of the gallbladder does not occur because the individual is too tense (the sympathetic nervous system being too present), the gallbladder is obstructed by gallstones, or if it has been removed, the intestine will be less alkaline and digestion of fat will consequently be less efficient, and therefore more energy-draining. We once again see that the balance of the ANS is responsible for many delicate functions. The small intestine secretes enzymes, mucus, water, and salt to optimize the digestive work in alkaline conditions.

Probiotics are these microorganisms that are often called 'good bacteria'. They reside in the intestine (some in the small intestine, others in the colon) and help us to break our food down into small, accessible particles. If the environment is acid, or after ingestion of antibiotics, which kill the intestinal flora, digestive problems will arise and an imbalance between the 'good' and the 'bad' bacteria will possibly occur.[4]

WASTING STORAGE PHASE (UNCONSCIOUS AND INVOLUNTARY)
In the large intestine, everything that has not been digested is concentrated and stored. Water and electrolytes are reabsorbed.

RECTAL PHASE (CONSCIOUS AND INVOLUNTARY OR VOLUNTARY)
Distension triggers the defecation reflex.

How do I lose my energy?
Following my personal observations and the testimonials of many patients, the following are some hypotheses that can explain the energy imbalance related to our body's requirements in terms of oxygen and hydrogen. Most of the hypotheses being advanced are related to the notions addressed in this chapter and in the previous chapter – which would render the task easier for you if you want to use them to form your own hypotheses, discuss them with your doctor and, find your own solutions that are adapted to your strengths and weaknesses. I have also compiled, in tables, certain vitamin and mineral deficiencies that you will find in Appendix 2. They are not exhaustive, but offer an interesting overview.[5]

HYPOTHESIS 1: LACK OF BREATHING EFFICIENCY AND AIR POLLUTION
I am stressed and my breathing is less abdominal than before. The stuffy air that I breathe in the city and in certain environments (office towers, newly paved streets, disinfected premises, etc.) lowers the efficiency of my cerebral oxygenation, makes my body react to polluting substances and perhaps even makes me anxious. In the evening, my nose is often blocked (especially in the city) and I often breathe through my mouth when I sleep.

HYPOTHESIS 2: MALABSORPTION OF LIPIDS

When my stomach is lacking hydrochloric acid, when it must be in an acid environment to help it break down the food I am absorbing into smaller elements, I digest less efficiently: it's the secondary effect that occurs when, for example, I take antacids when I have heartburn. Furthermore, my stomach loses its antiseptic armour against certain external organisms that the hydrochloric acid would have eliminated under normal conditions.[6] A drop in hydrochloric acid in the stomach is associated with an inflammation of the stomach wall.

I don't absorb my food very well because, since childhood, I have had trouble digesting fat. Is it possible that I have a fat-soluble vitamin deficiency (see Appendix 2C)? Could it be a result of a bad peristaltic rhythmic activity, which influences the acid-based balance of the digestive system? Or is it possible that the increasingly high volume of waste in my liver is forming amalgams with noncalcified bile salts, which could be the cause of my very high bile secretion and the abdominal pains under my ribcage? When the bile leaves my gallbladder during the digestive process, I have vertigo and this alkaline liquid tends to find itself in my stomach.[7]

HYPOTHESIS 3: PARASITIC INVASION IN AN
ACID INTESTINAL ENVIRONMENT

The refined food that I absorb acidifies my digestive tube. The pH in my intestinal flora is then imbalanced and becomes acid in my large intestine. Acidity is necessary as an antibacterial barrier in the stomach, but the rest of the digestive tube requires an alkaline environment to effectively absorb essential nutrients. This acidifying imbalance stimulates the proliferation of disease-causing microorganisms, like *Candida albicans*,[8] which intoxicates me.[9] My digestive system becomes a battleground on which undesirable parasites are at odds with the defensive arsenal of my digestive system which, as a result, can no longer send new anti-inflammatory troops without damaging the intestinal wall. This wall is not made for toxic residue left by these undesirable parasites. The waste resulting from the fermenting of this toxic cocktail creates an inflammation, the source of the abdominal pain. This gastric overload that allows excessively large molecules to travel from the stomach to the intestine, helps accentuate the proliferation of this undesirable bacteria. It is now recognized that taking antibiotics destroys the intestinal flora and constitutes a factor in the proliferation of *Candida albicans* and in the weakening of the digestive system.[10]

TABLE 5.2 Symptoms of chronic candidiasis compared to adrenal fatigue and magnesium deficiency symptoms[11]

ADRENAL FATIGUE	MAGNESIUM (MG) DEFICIENCY	CHRONIC CANDIDIASIS
PSYCHOLOGICAL SYMPTOMS		
Lack of concentration Forgetfulness Decreased mental clarity Irritability Decreased productivity Mental confusion when rushed	Irritability Decreased productivity Nervousness	Lack of concentration Forgetfulness Mental slowness Irritability Bipolar disorder/delusions (in extreme cases)
Inability to tolerate stress Anxiety/fears Feeling of despair	Less resistance to stress Depression	Depression
PHYSICAL SYMPTOMS		
Headaches: frequent and often unexplained Sudden lack of energy Persistent fatigue Trouble sleeping	Premature aging Persistent fatigue: decreased cellular metabolism and ATP transformation	Headaches Persistent fatigue
Brown spots on the face, neck and/or shoulders	More prone to cavities Brittle nails	
Sensitivity to cold Hypotension Dizziness Lack of consciousness Arrhythmia/palpitations Shortness of breath	Myocarditis Link with atherosclerosis Coronary lesions Tachycardia	Cold hands and feet Dizziness
Swollen lymph nodes (in the neck) Auto-immune diseases More prone to respiratory tract infections	Decreased phagocytosis Inflammation Oxydation Decreased resistance to diseases and infections More prone to respiratory tract infections	Nasal congestion Sinus problems Decreased resistance to diseases and infections

Difficulty digesting	Lack of appetite	Bad breath
Salt cravings	Nausea	Difficulty digesting
Weight loss	Vomiting	Indigestion
	Decreased bile secretion	Sugar and bread (yeast)
	Decreased pancreatic and	cravings
	intestinal secretions	Heartburn
		Belching
		Bloating
		Abdominal pain
		Constipation
		Diarrhea
		Rectal itching
Amplified premenstrual	PMS	Prostatitis
syndrome (PMS) (10 days)	Painful uterine contractions	Recurrent vaginal yeast
Decreased sexual desire	Responsible for renal stone	infections
	formation	
	Contributes to prostatic	
	adenoma	
Tremors when uptight	Tremors:	
Swollen ankles at night	• spasmophilia	
Agitated limbs	• tetanus	
Muscle weakness	Oedema	
	Muscle cramps	
	Numbness	
	Tingling sensation	
	Muscle weakness	
ASSOCIATED CONDITIONS		
Allergy exacerbation	Allergies and intolerances	Allergies
Multiple chemical	– due to reduced	Multiple chemical
sensitivities	phagocytosis	sensitivities
Respiratory diseases	Associated with modern	Weakened immune system
Rheumatoid arthritis	diseases	Development of immune
Fibromyalgia	Decreased resistance to	and auto-immune diseases
Other immune and auto-	stress	
immune disorders		

I suffer from flatulence, diarrhoea and heartburn. The lack of enzymes and probiotics and, jointly, the occurrence of harmful microorganisms, possibly result in exacerbation of known and unknown food intolerances whose process intensifies the imbalance. In Table 5.2, you can review another comparison between several medical conditions. We can easily see the relationships that exist between the different nutritional imbalances. It should be noted that chronic candidiasis is not a diagnosis in Western medicine.

HYPOTHESIS 4: FAST FOOD AND TOXICITY[12]

All sorts of additives, seasonings, trans and rancid fats, food colouring, sugars, and preservatives are found in fast-food restaurant food and in large-scale prepared dishes. Science considers reactions of intolerance to these products to be pseudo-allergies because, although they can trigger an inflammatory process, no antibodies are produced (immunoglobulin-IgE) against these substances. Inflammatory reactions are rather the result of the secretion of substances such as histamine and tyramine.

There are many undesirable molecules in the water I drink that overload the cellular maintenance mechanisms of my organism. I react to these toxins and to this accumulation of undesirable molecules. In other words, I fill my carburettor with impure gas and my engine fails! My cells lack fuel (hydrogen ions) to bind themselves to the available oxygen, and this imbalance rusts my cellular engine. In the 1970s it was realized that there were traces of aspirin in our waterways. Knowing that the most commonly prescribed medications are beta-blockers for coronary patients, antidepressants, and contraceptive hormones, it's possible that these products and other medical residues, as well as domestic and industrial products, are found, indirectly through the water and food that I eat, in my body–mind.[13]

Other substances consumed in excessive quantities have an adverse effect on the absorption of essential nutrients and encumber the digestive process. Trans fatty acids are particularly known for using enzymes that would normally be used by good fats in the production of cellular membranes and of the myelin of the nervous system. They increase the rate of LDL in the blood ('bad cholesterol'), lower the rate of HDL ('good cholesterol'), and increase the rate of Lp(a), a lipoprotein that is also associated with certain cardiac and cerebrovascular diseases. They are so harmful that the Canadian Parliament adopted a resolution to prohibit their usage in food products.[14]

HYPOTHESIS 5: PRODUCTION OF AN INFLAMMATORY HORMONE: PROSTAGLANDIN 2 (PGE2)

I consume many products from the animal kingdom and I therefore produce more arachidonic acid, which causes the production of prostaglandin PGE2 (eicosanoid hormone). This hormone is the main pathological inflammatory route, because its mediator is the enzyme cyclooxygenase-2 (COX-2),[15] which can trigger excessive inflammations – as opposed to prostaglandins PGE1 and PGE3 which are the inflammatory protection routes of the body against invaders.[16] For example, non-steroid anti-inflammatory drugs used to counter the inflammatory process of rheumatoid arthritis, among other things, have an inhibiting effect on the action of the COX-2 enzyme.[17]

HYPOTHESIS 6: DECREASED ESSENTIAL CHEMICAL REACTIONS

My diet is low in nutrients – vitamins and minerals, among other things. Consequently, harmony isn't always achieved in the steps involved in digesting and absorbing food. I may lack vitamins and rich phytochemicals because I don't each much fruit in the winter,[18] certainly not the five to ten portions of fruit and vegetables (more vegetables than fruit), as recommended by Canada's Food Guide. In addition, even in healthy food among our local products, I lack certain nutrients (see Appendix 2). As a result, my cellular motor fails because it lacks the enzymes or cofactors needed to create the necessary adequate chemical reactions when animal starch is transformed into glucose. There are possibly other substances whose beneficial effects are still overlooked or unknown by science that I am also missing.

HYPOTHESIS 7: FOOD INTOLERANCES

Food intolerances weaken my intestines and magnify the inflammatory process (which is already a big stress in itself): as a result, the intestines become porous to larger molecules,[19] which cause all sorts of toxins and trans fats to penetrate which do not ordinarily enter a healthy body in as large a volume. My body must then take on a greater role in cleaning the toxins, which is another overload for the entire organism. When you say allergy and invasion of the body, what you're actually saying is secretion of histamine and other substances that produce inflammation. This phenomenon is called *irritable bowel syndrome*, or worse, *leaky gut syndrome*. It's as if there were holes from my gas tank leading into my motor. I should therefore expect breakdowns.

HYPOTHESIS 8: THE CELLULAR DOOR IS PARTIALLY CLOSED

Because of a high level of stress over an excessively long period of time, my cells' locks no longer recognize the key of glucose molecules which penetrate them and also do not enable these molecules to supply them as fuel. They block the entry of glucose molecules, which means that they have become resistant to glucose to protect themselves against excessive oxidation: as the brain cells are the biggest consumers of glycolic energy, they are the first to demonstrate signs indicating a lack of fuel. An imbalance exists in the control of the level of blood and intracellular sugar: it is cortisol and insulin that are responsible for the balance in the sugar rate. Cortisol is responsible for maintaining the balance of the blood sugar level and insulin makes it penetrate the cells (see Chapter 13). My adrenal glands and my pancreas tire mutually. I suffer from hypoglycaemia. Since my muscles are badly nourished, they do not produce energy effectively, known as being 'in an aerobic phase', and create too much waste. They become very quickly and abnormally stiff, and the pain triggered by this stiffness is more intense than what I am used to.

HYPOTHESIS 9: ABUSE OF CELLULAR ENERGY FACTORIES

The energy manufacturing plants at the cellular level are damaged, and are therefore less effective for creating energy inside the cells. We even tend to think that a mutation could have affected them – for example, in people suffering from myalgic encephalomyelitis.

When certain chemical components in our body lose an electron, they are called *free radicals* or *oxidants*. These components move around freely in our body while 'stealing' electrons from other cells. The cellular damage occurs when the body lacks hydrogen ions, even if it has enough oxygen. The cells in the body become oxidized, in the same way that oxygen causes iron to rust. This oxidization damages the cellular DNA, hence the name oxidants. The damage created by the free radicals in the human body are what cause aging – premature or otherwise.

A success story of modifying food habits

Mary-Jane came to see me when she had been on disability for five months. To the extent that I explained the concept of energy from a cellular level and the food that we consume to create this energy, she changed certain habits, including those related to diet (cutting down on refined carbohydrates). She started shopping at a health food store near her house. As she suffered from cramps, burning, and abdominal bloating daily, she decided to take a combined probiotic supplement for the small intestine and the large intestine. In less than three months the distension and discomfort disappeared as well as the alternating diarrhoea and constipation. After four months of occupational therapy treatments, in which the Padovan Method® and the PCPSP programme were used, and sessions with a psychologist, Mary-Jane successfully went back to her energy-draining work environment. She can't change jobs right now, but has good tools for better managing the stressors in her environment. Physically, she uses better nutrients to produce the fuel she requires to cope with her daily adversity. Psychologically, she has learned to deal with her work environment with a different state of mind.

All these hypotheses, alone or combined, can result in direct or indirect energy inefficiency in the *Krebs Cycle*, which occurs within each mitochondrion of each cell in our body. Would some of these hypotheses be highly relevant in explaining your *persistent fatigue*?

Improving digestive harmony

Toxicity to the brain due to certain foods, bacterial invasion
and lack of proper nutrients, is shown more and more in
research to be linked to mental illness. This toxicity impairs
the efficiency of chemical reactions in the brain.

Absorption of nutrients is essential to your healing process. Just as in the performance of a talented violinist, rhythm and tempo must be respected in digestion to achieve consistency and coordination of the various digestive functions. If the strings are out of tune as a result of an unbalanced nervous system, the musician needs to tune them to ensure that they vibrate at the proper frequency. If the musician wants his instrument (his body–mind) to stay vibrant, it is his responsibility to cherish it and sustain it in an environment that is not abnormally stressful and exhausting for the mind, and that is not excessively alkaline, or too acid for the body. Furthermore, he must avoid creating an environment prone to mildew. If his musical repertoire is too narrow, he will limit his performance abilities.

Food intolerance and allergies

Intolerance can be caused by an enzyme deficiency (as in the case of milk that a person cannot digest due to a lack of the lactase enzyme), which triggers an inflammatory response but without creating antibodies. Allergy is an abnormal immunological response, that is, an inflammatory response with antibody production. Some scientists accept the hypothesis according to which a part of the population is becoming allergic to the things to which it is the most exposed. The following are the most common food intolerances and allergies in North America:

- milk and other milk products, especially fermented ones
- wheat
- all sources of gluten
- corn
- food additives (monosodium glutamate (MSG), food colouring, butylated hydroxytoluene (BHT)…)
- eggs
- stimulants: chocolate, coffee, tea and drinks containing guanine
- refined sugars and flours
- food containing histamine (eggs, chocolate, cheeses, fermented drinks, tomatoes, spinach, shellfish, fish…).

Milk intolerance

It was when I started eating more dairy products during my second pregnancy that I realized that these products were giving me terrible migraines lasting for 30 to 48 hours, and made a comeback barely 12 to 15 hours later. I had never had such long-lasting and incapacitating migraines. They stopped as soon as I eliminated milk and all dairy products from my diet.

Take stock of your food intolerances (which are possibly allergies) and systematically avoid them for at least three weeks, or even better, six months.[20] With respect to severe allergies (some resulting in anaphylactic shock), it is obvious that total abstinence is in order. Blood tests can reveal the presence and source of certain allergies (coeliac disease, a gluten allergy, is hereditary, while intolerance to wheat is not).

To do your investigative work, consult with a nutritionist, a naturopath, an allergist, or other health professional who knows a lot about food and environmental intolerances and allergies. If you lack the financial means, buy a book on the subject or visit a website based on scientific evidence.[21]

Many physicians advocate a method of disintoxication and also indicate the way of reintroducing the different foods according to a specific schedule, by avoiding the same food for four consecutive days to avoid any aggravation of allergy symptoms.[22] It is preferable that you are assisted in this process by a physician who is well versed in the field.

While you wait to find the right practitioner, totally avoid the foods to which you are sure to be allergic or intolerant. Don't take any risks with allergies.

Certain allergies and intolerances are with us for life. However, with the help of a medical follow-up, certain foods to which you are highly intolerant could eventually be reintegrated under medical supervision. With respect to intolerances, reintegrate the problematic foods by following the four-day rotation diet. This method can yield good results for disciplined people who do not cheat over four days.

If you are among those people who have severe allergic reactions or go into anaphylactic shock or suffer from severe inflammatory reactions, don't try this experiment unsupervised! Be responsible! Some reactions can be fatal!

Food intolerance and inflammation

By reducing the stressors in my diet through the above-described method, supervised by my doctor, I was successful in reducing the inflammation of the digestive tube and was then able to effectively absorb my food. I had to eliminate all dairy products (cow, goat, and sheep products), corn, wheat, monosodium glutamate, chocolate, and several other products. I needed two years to be able to successfully eat everything again – except milk – by following the rules set out in this section. If I stray from the rules, the inflammation returns with a vengeance. I recently learned that a brother and a sister of my father had been intolerant to milk since childhood.

Hypoglycaemia

If you are not sure you have symptoms of hypoglycaemia, go to the Hypoglycaemia Support Foundation website to inquire.[23] In the comparative table in Appendix 2, you will find the main signs of hypoglycaemia.[24]

If you have symptoms of reactive hypoglycaemia, it is important that you avoid sweet and refined foods, sugar substitutes, and fruits with a high concentration of sugar, especially dried fruits (which are full of sulphites and, as a result, tend to be highly allergenic).

Don't wait until you're hungry or for a craving to strike before you eat. Have more frequent, smaller meals. If you are severely affected, calculate approximately the same quantity of protein and complete carbohydrates during meals and snacks to slow down the speed at which carbohydrates are absorbed. The 'one third protein to two thirds complete carbohydrates' ratio is what is recommended by nutritionists to achieve a balanced diet, which is nevertheless not enough for some of my patients. For long-term effectiveness, it seems that the best proteins are rich in chlorophyll, such as spirulina and chlorella:[25] these two algae contain approximately 60 per cent protein, in addition to being rich in other essential nutrients.

Possible low glucose level 1

Alan, who has suffered from myalgic encephalomyelitis for six years, told me during a session that for many years prior to finding out that he was sick, he suffered from tremors during the night and, to calm them, went to the fridge to look for something to eat. His wife thought he was a glutton!

If you think you are going to solve your problem by consuming a sugar substitute, such as aspartame, you are mistaken: this substance is a stressor (even toxic) for your body and your level of insulin and cortisol will rise, then fall, leaving your cells with an even more significant lack of glucose.[26] Avoid foods with a *high glycemic index* and choose foods with a *low glycemic index.*[27]

Possible low glucose level 2

For more than six months I had to get up in the night to eat in order to lessen the stress related to malabsorption, even despite the fact that I would have a snack before going to bed and four meals a day with dietary supplements and snacks every two hours. I didn't even gain a single gram of weight!

According to Philpott and Kalita, 'low and high blood sugar can be evoked by foods of all types, whether fats, carbohydrates or proteins, and chemicals such as petrochemical hydrocarbons and even tobacco equally evoke abnormal sugar level curves in susceptible persons'.[28] This suggests that stress, *in all its forms*, stimulates the secretion of insulin, which can lead to *reactive hypoglycaemia*. These same authors specify that they have drawn up a list of several people, among those who were tested for their level of glycaemia using a 'glucose tolerance test' (GTT), of which the results announced diabetes within the first couple of hours following their test to then show a result of hypoglycaemia several hours after.[29] It therefore seems difficult to obtain a reliable hypoglycaemia test.

Diabetes or hypoglycaemia?

The GTTs that I took during my two pregnancies lasted three hours while the AHQ[30] recommends a five-hour GTT, precisely to properly diagnose hypoglycemia. Is it possible that the diabetes that was diagnosed during my first pregnancy was possibly a hypoglycemia warning sign that my body, which was already in a state of energy imbalance, was sending me?

Food supplements

Many doctors have come to the conclusion that supplementing our regular diet with vitamins and other nutrients is now necessary to maintain health and proper chemical reactions in our body.

It is clear that if you have severe malabsorption problems, you will show symptoms of a dietary deficiency (see Appendix 2). However, before taking supplements, the first thing you need to do is change your eating habits. This will cost you less money than supplements – while being effective. Food contains tens of thousands of phytochemicals whose benefits are incredible. For example, curcumin from turmeric and epigallocatechin-3-gallate from green tea, as described by Dr Béliveau, are only a very small part of the nutrients not found in a supplement.[31] These are molecules with major benefits for our body. It is therefore important that we change our eating habits, diversify our diet, and understand, once and for all, that there are energizing foods and energy-draining foods (consult Table 5.1). When you are functioning at less than 40 per cent of your energy potential, it is imperative that you cut down on any needless or energy-draining energy expense and change your eating habits to provide yourself with the phytochemicals used in the self-healing process. This is the best way to clear your energy debt.

If you are in need of vitamins, such as vitamin C, complex B group, and vitamin E (not only the inexpensive d-alpha-tocopherol), make sure, if you have intolerances, that you choose a hypoallergenic product. Look for pharmacies specializing in these products, and seek advice from professionals who are familiar with natural products. Certain health food stores also have astonishingly qualified staff and sell high-quality products.

Don't accept the first response as being the only response and the right one. If you opt for glandular extracts[32] – thyroid gland, adrenal glands, thymus – or for hormones that are so-called 'natural' or in a homeopathic form,[33] seek a doctor's supervision. If you have serious absorption problems, eat more frequently and in smaller quantities. This will enable you to avoid deficiencies, and will not put undue strain on your digestive system.

Some minerals can be very important when you are in the phase in which you are losing your nutrients as a result of frequent diarrhoea. Enzymes and probiotics are also useful in facilitating digestion and absorption. In addition, some of them will help you to evacuate the parasites that can infest your digestive tube by regulating and stabilizing your bowel movements.

When purchasing your probiotics, you need to keep in mind that certain products target the small intestine while others target the large intestine: ask questions to determine your specific needs. As you want to buy a living product,[34] look for products stored in the refrigerator in stores, rather than on the shelves, in the event that you are not guided by a professional. A good indicator of quality – and, unfortunately, of price also – are the companies that specialize in hypoallergenic products. The identification of human microflora is also a reliable indicator of a product's quality. Seek information from qualified professionals. Everyone has their own needs, based on their diet, sensitivity in terms of their organs and genetic baggage. What is fine for one person can be toxic for someone else. Consult and ask questions!

I won't give you the list of supplements that made me feel better at different points of my rehabilitation. Without them, the state of my health definitely would have weakened further. Once my body started to absorb food effectively and once my hypoglycaemia symptoms disappeared, I gradually reduced the vitamins, enzymes, and minerals. I needed two years to rebuild functional intestines. Since that time, I only use the probiotics and a few compounds intended to be taken daily. If it happens, on occasion, that I take supplements, it is based on my energy needs, on the quantity of food that I absorb, on the intensity of my physical activities, and on the bio-psycho-social stress that I have to manage. In other words, we need to increase our consumption of supplements from time to time, based on the circumstances that affect us.

I definitely benefited in several ways from certain supplements but these benefits were specific to me and are not necessarily the same for everyone. My health improved dramatically as a result of certain homeopathic products. (Paradoxically, before noting a decrease in symptoms, there was often an aggravation. This is why I don't believe it was a placebo effect.) In my quest to find a doctor, I had to consult several homeopaths and naturopaths before finding someone who understood the interrelational aspect of the body, that is, who worked according to the PNI perspective. I will describe the benefits I experienced after taking magnesium (however, you need to keep in mind the following facts).

Physiological stress increasing inflammation

When I engaged in an intense physical activity (greater than 10 METS) during the months in which I had a short menstrual cycle (which ended, possibly because of a lack of progesterone after ovulation), I would be putting so much stress on my body that my digestive system would start to burn with acid, without any other triggering stressors being present. My entire digestive tube was affected. In other words, my digestive system's inflammatory reaction seemed to be related to physiological stress other than that coming from the food I was eating!

The importance of magnesium

- Magnesium is needed for several hundred chemical reactions in our body.

- Approximately 70 per cent of the American population suffer from a magnesium deficiency.[35]

- Calcium cannot penetrate the bones without magnesium.

- Magnesium is an excellent muscle relaxant. It lessens muscle and menstrual cramps: it is therefore useful to take just before and during your period.[36] With zinc and vitamin B6, a magnesium deficiency is one of the nutritional deficiencies that possibly causes restless leg syndrome, sometimes referred to as 'jimmy legs', which is so common in exhausted people.[37]

- Intramuscular and intravenous injections of magnesium in the form of modified Myers' cocktail yield good results in people suffering from various syndromes related to persistent fatigue.[38]

- Research shows that a magnesium deficiency is very common in people suffering from myalgic encephalomyelitis.[39] However, other research exists that does not indicate any evidence of a magnesium deficiency.[40]

- A lack of magnesium is associated with metabolic syndrome (insulin resistance syndrome or syndrome X). This metabolism anomaly prevents the body from responding normally to insulin, which creates an imbalance effect on the cellular glucose and the production of energy.[41]

- Some reasons to increase your magnesium consumption when you experience symptoms of a deficiency (see Table 5.3).

  ○ North American soil,[42] is magnesium-deficient. Therefore, as a result, some of us tend to be more magnesium-deficient, especially in periods of high stress, with all the repercussions that this deficiency can have on our health (see Appendix 2). The more stress there is, the more intensely the Krebs cellular mill turns to bring available energy to the system – and this cycle needs magnesium to work properly.

  ○ As in North America, Australia's soils are also depleted of magnesium.[43]

  ○ The industrial refining of grain, the food preservation methods, and the food processing and preparation methods deprive us of magnesium.

  ○ The hyperactive and reckless lifestyle of modern life demands a greater use of magnesium for the different cellular functions.

  ○ Calcium helps muscles to contract and magnesium helps muscles to relax. It is estimated that our ancestors had in their diet a calcium/magnesium ratio of 1:1. The current North American ratio is 15:1.[44]

  ○ In Europe, the average daily magnesium intake is less than the minimum daily requirement for many countries, with figures for Finland and the UK particularly poor.[45]

Magnesium is naturally found in the food we consume, in dried fruits (preferably without nitrites), in nuts, green vegetables, complete grains (unrefined), dairy products, certain fruits such as berries, figs, and avocados, and in red meats such as beef and lamb.

Magnesium supplements are available in different forms based on people's individual needs. Before starting this type of treatment, you should be followed by a doctor who is familiar with magnesium or who shows an open mind to magnesium as a treatment option and who is ready to assist you. *Not everyone who suffers from persistent fatigue is necessarily magnesium-deficient; use judgement and observe your symptoms.*

In my case, my blood magnesium level fell within the average, but on the lower end. The blood test does not reflect the intracellular magnesium level.[46] I tried many types of magnesium supplements based on my state of health and my menstrual cycle. They ended up being very useful, as I describe below – I won't, however, give the doses, because they vary from one individual to another, based on each individual's problems.[47]

- In tablet form, before a meal, magnesium calmed my tremors and brought me the minimum energy I needed to carry out my basic daily activities, when I was bedridden. My digestive system wasn't absorbing nutrients well, which forced me to eat five to seven times a day, in addition to having a night-time snack.

- In powder form, with Complex B vitamins, at the beginning of naturopathic and homeopathic treatments, magnesium especially reduced my constant pain and hypoglycaemia.

- Sublingual liquid solutions caused restless leg syndrome to disappear, which kept me up sometimes at night. The syndrome disappeared in under 15 minutes. The solutions also lessened my menstrual cramps.

- When my doctor suggested that I take intramuscular injections of magnesium and vitamin B12, I took the time to find out about possible side effects, and then agreed to take it while being careful not to take the two substances at the same time, so I could experience the effects of each one. The magnesium injection is relaxing, both for the muscles and the blood vessels. I had to take them lying down because my blood pressure, which was already low, dropped even more a few minutes after the injection. In two or three minutes, the pains that I had felt constantly for months disappeared within a few hours; later, they disappeared over a few days, and then all together. Since magnesium is a relaxant and facilitates sleep, I had to take a nap when I got home: this is why I preferred to receive the injections at the end of the day. The doctor also had to adjust the dose downward.

- Still today and as needed, I take a magnesium supplement before intense physical activity – otherwise, my legs start dancing before I go to bed. I also take it during the first three days of my period, which spares me from severe menstrual pain (the pain reappears when I forget to take the supplement) and, often, spares me from a migraine.

It is important to get the proper information before taking a supplement. It is, among other things, not recommended to take magnesium if you suffer from kidney failure, intestinal obstruction, abnormally low heartbeat, or from *myasthenia gravis*.[48] If you take medication, ask your pharmacist about its possible interactions with magnesium.

Summary

Developing useful habits breaks us free from obsolete habits and addictions of all kinds.

1. Go for a walk outside, when possible, after a meal. Gravity and light physical activity facilitate digestion.

2. Avoid spicy foods if you are sensitive to them. However, remember that several spices, such as turmeric and the garlic–cayenne pepper mixture, have indisputable anticancerous, anti-inflammatory, antibacterial and antioxidant properties.

3. Drink water, if possible of good quality;[49] many people believe that they are hungry when, in fact, they are thirsty. Once again, it is important to find a balance: too much or not enough water increases the stress imposed on our body. Avoid drinking during or just after a meal so as not to force your food bolus out the door before it is absorbed. Adding a little lemon or lime juice to water enhances digestion as well as liver and gallbladder functions.

4. Avoid eating and drinking from plastic and polystyrene containers.[50]

5. Look for alkaline rather than acidating foods.

6. Consume five to ten portions of fruit and vegetables per day (more vegetables than fruit).

7. Use necessary medication. Avoid medication that is not necessary: it puts excessive strain on the liver, whether prescribed or available over the counter. Colouring and preservatives added to the pills can also be harmful to those who are hypersensitive. Some pharmacies specialize in compounding preparations when this type of problem arises.[51]

8. Avoid alcohol: it lowers vitamin absorption; it is toxic for the liver and can contain an allergenic substance – in addition to being a depressant that you don't need. Alcohol and benzodiazepines (discuss these with your doctor) are related to GABA receptors. Their calming effect only lasts a short while and they need to be taken in increasingly greater quantities for the same small relief of stress to be felt, because they desensitize the receptors and reduce them in quality.[52] The risk of addiction is high.

9. If you take nutritional supplements to foster your healing, make sure you are followed by a competent professional. Like medication, these products can contain colouring or an ingredient to which you may be intolerant; vitamin C, for example, is often prepared from corn. Absorbing an excessively high dose of a product, even if it is good, is as exhausting for the liver and the digestive system as is a deficiency. This is especially important for non-hydrosoluble vitamins.

10. Take care of your liver and your gallbladder. Consult with a specialist, especially if you suspect the presence of gallstones. These can be detected on an ultrasound.

11. Follow the second exercise in Chapter 8 to promote parasympathetic digestive harmony.

You have a power, which is that of managing the energy that you consume and the way in which you consume it. Overconsumption, just like choosing foods devoid of nutritional value, is energy-draining, while eating in a balanced manner, in a reasonable timeframe, facilitates the digestive process and is energizing. It is your responsibility to make informed choices to restore your energy mill.

Chapter 6
Energy: What Is It?

Energy is power.

From the basic concepts learned in school, I remember that *everything contains energy*, whether in the form of work, kinetic, or potential energy. From the pebble to the most sophisticated multicellular organism, everything contains energy. Let's also remember that 'Nothing is lost, nothing is created; everything transforms itself.' According to the famous equation, $E = mc^2$, mass is also a form of energy.

The discoveries of the last few decades about cells and subatomic particles demonstrate that these particles contain minuscule energy units. This has given rise to a new wave of research leading us to a model that assumes that life has an electromagnetic component and that it cannot be explained only by mechanical and biochemical means.

Physical vibrations
Vibrations picked up by the senses

Our eyes, ears, skin, tongue, and nose have receptors that pick up well-defined waves. These receptors are specialized structures that convert different forms of energy, introduced by the outside world, into electrical energy.[1] Our senses are like radios that can receive only a small scope of information frequencies from the outside environment. For example, our eyes have sensors from a specific electromagnetic spectrum. Our senses therefore only impart to us a small part of the information pertaining to reality. Because you don't pick up the radio or cellular telephone waves doesn't mean that they don't exist; it is enough to humbly recognize our sensory limitations and intuitively realize that something else exists that influences our energy level.

Certain other receptors, in our joints, muscles, and vestibular system, work a little differently. They receive data on our position in space that stems from different parts of our body and that takes into account both the other body parts and the position of the body with respect to the earth. The force of gravity acts as a magnet pulling our body in its direction. It is the information picked up by the joints and vestibular sensors that teaches us about our position vis-à-vis what lies above and what lies below.

To the five senses with which we are so well acquainted, I will add the sense of life – or survival, depending on how we look at it. It is one of 12 senses proposed by the sensory model of the founder of anthroposophy, Rudolph Steiner. What's distinctive about this sense is that we are aware of it when things are not going well. These are the neurovegetative manifestations of an ANS in a state of alert. It is this sense that gives us the information when our digestion is not functioning smoothly, when we're feeling bloated, suffering from heartburn, and sense a general digestive sluggishness. It informs us about the physiological food being ingested, and sends this information to our nervous system. It also sends us information regarding non-physiological food: for example, in the form of bowel sounds and feverishness triggered by the excitement felt at a big evening event, or a knot in the stomach when bad news is suddenly announced or when we are in a situation in which we feel 'we can't take it anymore'. Basically, this sense is the physical manifestation of our emotional state. Unfortunately, despite the fact that it is a rich source of information, in our society we tend to suffocate it with antacid and anti-reflux medication, with antibiotics, anti-inflammatories, etc.

Basically, we can say that the only interaction used by the human body to communicate – that is, to receive and process information from the environment – is *electromagnetic* in nature (except for distinguishing between up and down, which is linked to gravity). It is this type of interaction that we resort to when we use energy at the cellular level (described in Chapter 4). With our senses alone, we are highly limited in our understanding of the universe. This is why we are continually inventing devices, namely, energy sensors. As such, we can better understand the universe in which we live.

All *energy* harnessed by the senses is *information* that our environment sends to our nervous system. We can therefore refer to it as info-energy.

This info-energy is carried through our body–mind by information messengers that are known as neurotransmitters (or neuropeptides) and hormones produced by the endocrine glands, the immune system and by other organs in our body. This info-energy consequently affects all the cells of our PNI super system. In Figure 6.1 you will see a diagram that roughly illustrates the impact of info-energy picked up by the senses and perceived by the body–mind as a threat or stressor – in the case, for example, of a bear appearing on a bicycle path while you're peacefully riding your bike.

Vibrations not picked up by the senses

All the objects in our daily life possess vibratory power. All living beings possess an energy field. Several scientists have hypothesized that the electrodynamic field discovered by Burr would be a so-called morphic or morphogenic field.[2] This morphic field would animate each organism or self-organized system. According to Sheldrake, it would be responsible for organizing and coordinating the components of the organism; it would preserve its integrity and would enable it to regenerate. It would organize everything: atoms, molecules, cells, and tissues of organisms, even ecosystems, societies, solar systems and galaxies. Some research suggests that before any illness there is a change, an incoherence in the individual's energy field, and we can detect this incoherence with sophisticated equipment.[3]

Fritz-Abert Popp[4] has reintroduced the term 'biophoton'[5] to describe a permanent luminous emission given off from every biological substance and that allows us to assess the state of coherence of living organisms. This luminous energy[6] that differs from thermal radiation cannot be seen by the naked eye but can be seen if sophisticated equipment is used. According to the theory, these biophotons would be stored in DNA molecules in which there would be a change on an energy level. This constant exchange of absorption and photonic emission would form a communication network between the cells, tissue, and organs inside the body.

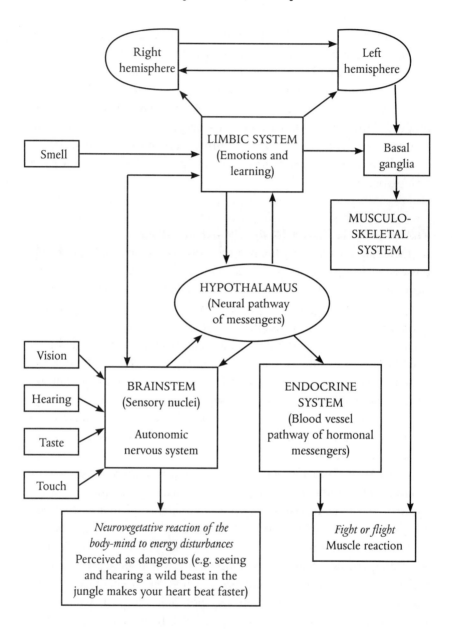

FIGURE 6.1 Reaction to the info-energy picked up
by our senses and perceived as a stressor

In his studies Dr Popp has made several observations on carcinogenic substances: they have trouble communicating, react only to a specific light wavelength and only respond to certain frequencies.[7] Different forms of stress, and even the phenomenon of aging to which oxidation is associated at the cellular level, due to increased stress, increase the rate of photonic emissions.[8] Even the food that we consume could have an impact on our electromagnetic coherence. We actually see that the best food for one's health would emit the weakest and most consistently intense light.[9]

Dr Masaru Emoto photographed water in a crystal form at the freezing point while he exposed it to the influence of different music (from Beethoven at one end of the spectrum to heavy metal at the other), emotions (from energizing to energy-draining), different names of people (from Mother Teresa of Calcutta to Hitler), etc. The images of water exposed to an energizing influence reveal a highly structured organization of crystals, and comparatively deformed and disorganized crystals form when energy-draining stimuli appear.[10] According to Dr Emoto,[11] water reacts differently to these stimuli, and this reaction could be similar where we are concerned, since we are composed primarily of water… Here again, the organizational coherence of certain forms of energy takes centre stage.

According to Traditional Chinese Medicine (TCM), which has been in existence for several millennia, the body contains 'vital energy (qi)' pathways, called 'meridians'. These meridians were scientifically shown by Hiroshi Motoyama and were later confirmed by other researchers.[12] Most meridians have a name based on certain key organs. In Western society we are only beginning to scientifically prove the benefits of certain categories of TCM treatments reflected in vital energy,[13] including the stimulation effect of certain acupuncture points on brain activity by the use of magnetic resonance as a measuring instrument.[14]

For several decades Western medicine has been using the electromagnetic component of the body to make diagnoses and conduct research. If we accept the data yielded by magnetic resonance imaging (MRI), which gives us highly precise images, for diagnostic purposes, it is illogical to deny that this quantum aspect of the human body exists. Furthermore, other medical research demonstrates the benefits resulting from the use of single or repetitive transcranial magnetic stimulation on the brain of patients suffering from various conditions such as depression, migraine, and cerebral vascular accidents. The results prove that treatment favours the self-healing process.[15]

LOCATIONS AND CLIMATE

Jean Bricard discovered that 'micro pollutants suspended in the air, which acquire a negative charge, are eliminated'.[16] When the air only has a few negative oxygen ions, it is polluted (like during hot summer days, in big cities, where the air is filled with smog). When there is a profusion of negative oxygen ions, the air is healthy. In the mountains and in close proximity to the sea, the concentration of negative ions would increase the biofield (the biofield bears a negative load), while certain atmospheric conditions with a strong positive load decrease it.[17] Negative ions are found in high quantities in nature: by the sea, in the mountains, in the forest, and at the base of waterfalls. In the house, they are found under the shower. They are more plentiful in the country than in the city. Compelling data demonstrate these beneficial effects on people suffering from asthma, hay fever, high blood pressure, and heartburn. However, the possible benefits were not noted as significant on so-called 'normal' subjects.[18]

ELECTROMAGNETIC SMOG

The appliances that we use on a daily basis emit waves that flow through and influence our body. We are not yet aware of the long-term effects that many of these waves have on our health, but they affect us.[19] And even though we do not know how these waves work, science advises that we exercise caution.[20] We only have to think about the effects of X-rays on Marie and Pierre Curie or of the effects of nuclear radioactivity to intelligently use electromagnetic technology without abusing it. Since we all have a biofield or a morphic field full of information, it would be logical to expect it to be affected by a wave of information that flows through it.

Psychological vibrations

Everything that vibrates in the universe interferes with other vibrations; sometimes they cancel one another out, sometimes they amplify each other.

Emotions

People fuelled by energizing emotions who gravitate around us subjectively seem to make us vibrate – like when one plays the piano and the vibrations are transmitted to the nearby guitar. Our bodies also vibrate. It has been scientifically proven that we can feel what others feel: this is known as *emotional resonance*.[21] It is a tendency that is spontaneous, involuntary, and therefore unconscious. We synchronize our facial expressions with those of the people with whom we interact. Through our senses we pick up the emotions of others around us and our emotional molecules start vibrating all together.[22]

When we are in a vulnerable state, we quickly realize that surrounding energy-draining emotions have a draining effect on our emotional energy level. Undergoing an emotional shock, like a major scare when driving, a betrayal, a big disappointment, the death of someone close, drains us emotionally. These life experiences consequently produce changes in the PNI system and the ANS and weaken our immune defences. An energy-related weakness exists. It also affects our loved ones and the people with whom we interact in our daily lives.

Seeing an action movie or learning about the death of Princess Diana stimulates the sympathetic nervous system, which is tied to the emotions that cause us stress. Watching a documentary show on Mother Teresa can have an energizing subjective effect, even in subjects who have no interest in charity. Objectively, it boosts immunoglobulin A, an antibody that attacks colds. This is called the 'Mother Teresa Effect'.[23] Many research studies have revealed the presence of these PNI phenomena.[24]

Dr Pert describes peptides, the *molecules of emotions* of our body as having a vibratory and rhythmically dancing movement around the cells. Once it is in harmony with the cell, the molecule, like a key, enters the 'keyhole' of the selected cell to combine with it.[25] Peptides are the molecules that send information through our body. These peptides are the messengers of info-energy. Wherever information, coming from outside, arrives at our nervous system, by way of our senses, scientists find a strong concentration of receptors of neuropeptides.[26]

The mental component

We know that our behaviour is too quick to be initiated by our conscience. Well before having recognized language that is heard (at

400 msec), we recognized semantic information (at 200 msec). We react before information is transmitted by the brain's neurotransmitters and by hormones in the bloodstream. While seeking an explanation to this problem, where the speed by which information is spread is faster than all the known interneuron connections, Dr Karl Pribram developed a holographic model of the brain in which each part contains the whole. According to him, the perception is the result of a complex reading and a transformation of sensory information to which all the parts of the brain contribute. For him, as for other researchers, the processes in the brain would operate on a quantum level.

Thought would vibrate faster than the body and would not be confined to the body for sending and receiving information (info-energy). Thought would be a highway that is similar to the Internet route: based on the quality of our interface (of attention and receptiveness), we would have access, consciously or not, when we are awake or dreaming. In the same way that the Internet is a process that differs from that of the telephone in receiving information, the alpha brainwave, which is in correlation with a change in the state of consciousness – as during meditation – could be the way of accessing and being on the wavelength corresponding to a higher energy level than that of the usual waking state. This would therefore enable us to perceive reality differently. According to scientific researchers in this field, our brain would communicate with all the cells in our body by way of interferential waves. Perceiving an object would mean being in resonance with it, that is, by synchronizing us with it.[27] Here again, there is an essential element of coherence.

Extensive research is currently being conducted on the effects of intention (thought) on matter, two forms of energy that had historically been separated in the Western world, science studying matter and religion, thought.[28]

Social vibrations

According to quantum physics, everything in the universe is interconnected and intertwined. Since people are part of the universe, we follow the same rules even though our senses do not reflect that aspect of reality.

The relationships we have with others are very complex from an energy perspective. There is, first of all, the energy field of physical bodies that interact with one another, then the emotional component, whether it is conscious or unconscious. Certain researchers issue the hypothesis according to which even unknown thoughts of others and the beating hearts have a vibratory mode that influences us unbeknownst to ourselves! According to a study reported by Paul Pearsall, children who regularly eat their supper with their family, and sit at the same table at around the same time every day, tend to have fewer colds and other infections than those who do not enjoy the benefit of a regular boost of this subtle energy that life can bring.[29] Other studies emphasize a vibratory consistency between healers and their patients.[30]

There is currently a 'global conscience' project launched by Dr Dean Radin and his colleagues with the help of random number generators throughout the world. At spontaneous events such as the tsunami disaster or the destruction of the Twin Towers, these generators saw their results influenced by nonlocalized mental coherence, that is, by the widespread attention given to these events by a large part of the global population.

Spiritual vibrations

Studies reveal that independent of people's state of health, age or sex, those who pray regularly have a better state of mental health.[31] Other research demonstrates that only an intention can have remote repercussions. In other words, an intention can have effects that are felt on the other end of the planet.[32] What power do you have when you are told, for example, that the recovery rate of the illness from which you are suffering is 5 per cent? Are you going to believe that you are part of those 5 per cent or are you rather going to group yourself among the 95 per cent of people who do not overcome the illness and, thinking this way, perpetuate the belief in these deterministic statistics that belong to the past, while the present remains to be created? Why wouldn't we rather use *hope* and our convictions like a placebo in our health system, rather than the *nocebo (negative placebo)* of statistics, prognoses, and scientific dogma that are limited to perceptions that do not take into consideration a more complete set of data?

Exercise 6.1: Indexing energy-draining and energizing stimuli

I have indexed here the energy-draining stimuli drawn from the experiences of people that I have treated, and have classified them based on each of the previously described dimensions. You can use these particular stimuli as food for thought in an effort to become aware of the occurrences that eat up your energy and those that enhance it. It is a good tool to use to learn how to avoid certain situations, when possible, and to have control over those contexts that cannot be avoided.

Spiritual vibrations: For most of my patients, contact with nature is described as a healthful state and even, in many patients, as a spiritual experience. Watching the evening news in which we are inevitably shown wars, genocides and other disasters is considered 'draining' because we often experience a feeling of powerlessness when faced with such atrocities.

Mind vibrations: For some, intensive intellectual reading over a long period and excessive 'consumption' of violent films or programmes containing aggressive subject matter are recognized energy-draining factors. Behaviours and thought patterns that trigger energy-draining emotional reactions are described as being exhausting. Certain meditation and taiji techniques are valued by my clients who realize the benefit they feel when they do not allow themselves to get carried away by the incessant flow of their energy-draining thoughts.

Sociocultural vibrations: Either consciously or unconsciously, exhausted people tend to avoid crowds. Some need to put up barriers and bridges between themselves and their employer, their spouse, their family... to be able to better survive and heal. Family harmony, a good supper among friends, a romantic date, in a nutshell, the friendliness with people we love and who respect us is felt as energizing.

Physical vibrations picked up by the senses: My clients suffering from migraines often complain of the odour emitted by tar and cleaning products (especially women and, even more frequently, cleaning women); some complain of symptoms of oestrogen dominance (see Appendix I). Among the most exhausted, I frequently observe aggressiveness when they find themselves in the presence of someone who wears perfume or who smokes (even when this person does not smoke in their presence: they are bothered by the smell of clothes that smell of cigarette smoke). Noise, certain types of music and bright lighting (such as those given off from a television, a computer, or a streetlamp outside a bedroom) make many people consciously react. Among individuals who are on disability leave from work and among seniors, the mobile phone vibrate mode is enough to make them uneasy, even if they are unable to articulate the specific reason as to why they are uncomfortable. People in relatively good health describe silence, affectionate caresses, classical music, the beauty of nature, and certain works of art as being comforting and soothing.

Physical vibrations not picked up by the senses: Some of my patients avoid neon-lit superstores but they are unable to say why these places drain them. Those who consume organic food more often notice a qualitative improvement in their energy level. It is recognized that ill people who have a pet reduce their risk of depression. Even caring for plants or a vegetable garden is felt as being energizing.

I advise those who feel they are undergoing an energy bankruptcy or are approaching such a state, to refer to Table 6.2 to create a coping tool. From the physical to the spiritual dimension of your life, note the vibrations that appear to you as energy draining or as energizing, in the two columns of Table 6.2. This will give you an idea of what to foster in your lifestyle and what to avoid. For those who are still able to work, but whose energy debt is starting to weigh on them, this exercise will represent a sound investment in vibrant healthy energy, which will reduce the interest on their mortgage.

This exercise is a tool designed to make us aware of the presence of energy-draining and energizing stimuli. Once the observation is made, it is easier to recognize, and consequently avoid, energy-draining stimuli when it is possible or to modify those stimuli that cannot be avoided in order to adopt a new outlook conducive to energizing stimuli. It is up to you to seek energizing rather than energy-draining effects. The sooner you initiate this exercise, the more you will preserve your energy for activities essential to your daily life – energy that will help you to regenerate the cells of your distressed organs.

TABLE 6.2 Effects of vibrations on vital energy

VIBRATIONS	ENERGY-DRAINING	ENERGIZING
SPIRITUAL		
PSYCHOLOGICAL		
SOCIOCULTURAL		
PHYSICAL		

Summary

If we adhere to the hypothesis and to scientific research that suggests that each of us possesses a biofield and that a breach forms in this field before a physiological illness arises, it would make sense to look into the problem when we feel some uneasiness or ailment, rather than naively masking it. It is healthy to find energizing alternatives and to avoid the tendencies we have to excessively exhaust our energy resources.

Emotional shocks, car accidents, and other violent physical trauma appear to disrupt the biofield. Other factors, for example, environmental toxicity or a former virus, also seem to contribute to destabilizing this field, and other environmental waves probably alter it. Many studies will be necessary in the future to gain a better understanding of these phenomena because we are still only in the early stages. Each of us has a responsibility to do our part while always maintaining a critical eye. It is up to each one of us to seek the help of reliable professionals, with whom we have no conflict of interest, who could guide us in the steps we need to take to achieve well-being.

Chapter 7

The Rhythms of Life

The only real men are those capable of delving into themselves,
their cosmic spirits capable of descending deep enough
to examine their relationships with the great universal rhythm.[1]

Robert Musil

Neurovegetative rhythms

The autonomous regulating functions of our body follow a rhythm. One of the main signs of derailment of the neurohormonal orchestration is the imbalance of the autonomous nervous system (ANS). The ANS presses its sympathetic accelerator pedal to the floor, and the parasympathetic braking system appears ineffective in countering this excess. This autonomous disturbance makes itself felt through a derailment of the neurovegetative rhythms. Imagine you just received some shocking news (positive or negative) and observe the repercussions of this announcement on your body–mind: your heart rate accelerates, you pant, your stomach contracts, you cry or laugh, etc.[2]

Breathing rhythm

When you rise in the morning, think of what a precious privilege
it is to be alive – to breathe, to think, to enjoy, to love.

Marc Aurelius

Our breathing cycle is very important for bringing good oxygenation to the cells in our body. Many people suffering from a psycho-neuro-immuno-endocrine (PNI) imbalance are going to feel out of breath. Some can even experience symptoms of a panic attack: they have trouble breathing and start hyperventilating. Others breathe through the mouth and/or use the upper abdomen (thoracic or rib breathing), which are superficial breathing patterns because the diaphragm can no longer recreate natural abdominal breathing, like that found in babies.[3]

Breathing is controlled by a voluntary nerve, namely, the phrenic nerve. It can therefore be consciously controlled and modified. However, if you try to hold your breath for a long time, you realize there is an involuntary, unconscious control that exists in this breathing that is regulated by the ANS. Science shows us that conscious respiratory rhythm has a modulating effect on the ANS and a direct effect on the parasympathetic nervous system.[4] The very fact of consciously observing one's breathing has a favourable impact on respiratory rhythm and therefore influences the ANS balance.

Each time you exhale, or engage in superficial thoracic breathing, as opposed to abdominal or lateral thoracic breathing at rest, an increased residue of stuffy air, which reduces the gas exchange during the subsequent inhalation, is left in the lungs.[5] It is as if you only half empty the dishwater from your sink after a meal and proceed to add clean water to the sink to wash the dishes from the following meal.

Nasal breathing allows inflowing air to ionize: the right nostril through which you breathe acquires a slightly more negative burden, and the left nostril becomes slightly more positive.[6] The air that penetrates a nostril activates the opposite hemisphere of the brain. Regularly (almost every 90 minutes), there is a natural tendency to lateralize the air flow, which has the effect of changing the *cerebral dominance*.[7]

Patient and sleep apnoea

John would describe himself as a person who has always been anxious. He is obese and has suffered from sleep disorders for many years. John breathes through his mouth. He has trouble breathing through his nose because of the ogival anatomical form of the hard palate and a congenital malformation (a malocclusion) of his lower jaw, which creates enormous stress on the joints in his jaw. I strongly suspected that he was suffering from bruxism (clenching and grinding of the teeth at night), which he confirmed to me. He suffered from repeated ear infections over the years, probably caused by the anatomical compression of his auditory tubes (cartilaginous ducts between the back of the ear and the middle ear, located above the hard palate) linked to the shape of his palate. During his occupational therapy exercises, John had trouble breathing through his nose. He was short of breath. When he lay on his stomach, he wasn't able to breathe through his nose, and when he did, his breathing became chaotic and he would start coughing every time he tried to fall asleep in the evening while lying in this position. I suggested that his doctor administer some tests on him in order to screen for sleep apnoea. The results confirmed my observations during therapy. Sleep apnoea contributes to the imbalance in ANS rhythms; it is therefore an additional risk factor for this man.

The air that enters through the nose moistens the nasal cavities and the larynx rather than parching them, while inhaling through the mouth has a dehydrating effect. Nasal breathing also heats the air that enters the body, which increases the effectiveness of the gas transfer occurring in the lungs. The cold air that enters through the nasal cavity and the sinuses effectively cools the largest consumer of energy in the body – the brain – because energy production consequently leads to dissipated heat. Breathing through the mouth does not allow energy to be optimized. Furthermore, it weakens the immune system because air is not filtered by the nasal passages, which permits penetration of undesirable particles that attack the tonsils (if one still has them) and the rest of the immune system. According to Padovan, breathing through the mouth would result in postural, esthetic, even psycho-emotional, alterations.[8] It is easy to extrapolate and to draw the conclusion that these alterations could burden our mind-body with other tensions.

The main muscles involved in breathing are the diaphragm, the abdominal, and the intercostal muscles. Other voluntary muscles are also involved in breathing, namely the large and small pectorals, the lateral muscles, and the neck flexors. All these muscles are controlled voluntarily.

Breathing is subcortically controlled by the brain in the brainstem by groups of neurons many of which are located in a region known as the *reticular formation*. Regulation of the breathing rhythm occurs at this level. Without going into detail, we can say that a group of neurons triggers inhaling or exhaling and another group controls the rate and pattern of breathing. The region sensitive to chemical changes in the brainstem contains neurons that receive information on the concentration of hydrogen ions (H+) formed by the CO_2 dissolved in the environment, and that regulate the rhythm and pattern of breathing to enable the body to maintain partial pressure of oxygen and carbon dioxide at constant values.[9] Peripheral receptors in the aorta also respond to gas changes. Controls in terms of breathing are closely related to the cardiovascular centre. An intimate relationship therefore exists between heart rate and breathing rhythm.

Most of the time, adjustments in rhythm are made unconsciously, but we can have a conscious influence on breathing through the cortical ramifications of the brain. Stretching receptors in the surface of the bronchial tubes and the lungs also have an influence on inhaling through the parasympathetic nervous pathways.

Cardiac rhythm

Our heart is a marvellous pump that beats at a systolic-diastolic rate between 64 and 80 times per minute at rest, on average, according to our physical condition. Its rhythm slightly resembles a triple meter (like a waltz). It also has its own unconscious pump regulator and can be consciously controlled, with a little training.[10] The autonomous control centre of the cardiac rhythm is also located in the brainstem.

The rhythms of digestion

To simplify, let's say that the rhythms of digestion constitute a set of functions that already develop in the mother's uterus and that are triggered by *suction* around the tenth week of gestation. *Suction* is a powerful rhythm that is already harmonized with the heart rate of the intrauterine (that of the foetus) and of the extrauterine (that of the mother). The facial muscles required for a baby to suck, to absorb food and liquid, and for an adult to kiss, have an effect on certain specific neurovegetative reactions. It is one of our body's critical functions that our society has often rejected for the sake of convenience (since the Second World War) while minimizing the following impacts:

- the importance of breast milk for immune system development

- the need for Omega-3 fat contained in breast milk, required for the myelinization of the baby's brain[11]

- the intimate relationship between a mother and baby and the entire emotional memory related to this function, stored in the limbic system

- the establishment of nasal breathing

- establishing proper coordination of the entire musculature of the mouth, the jaw, and the neck to ensure that the second and third rhythms related to the digestive process, i.e. chewing and swallowing function properly.[12]

In the Western world, the need to *chew* is rarely satisfied when we consume fast food and soft-textured food. We see a lot of children who chew on their pencils at school to soothe themselves, and many who bite their fingernails. People suffering from PNI disorder suffer from *bruxism* for different reasons. The rhythm at which we *chew* is more pronounced when we eat harder foods: crunching on nuts and chewing on a chicken bone or a veal chop has a soothing effect on the jaw muscles that carry out the work. The muscles relax after a more demanding session of chewing.

Swallowing, which appears in the thirteenth week intrauterine, is stimulated by *suction*, which makes the amniotic fluid enter the mouth and already stimulates the beginning of digestion. After swallowing, oesophageal peristalsis movements and the whole digestive process get under way in a rhythmic fashion. To be able to swallow, we have to stop breathing, allowing time for the food bolus to pass, while preventing it from partially penetrating the airways. All these functions are closely tied to and controlled by the brainstem structures. In Chapter 12, you will find suggested methods for relaxing the perioral muscles and reestablishing some of its rhythms.

We also know that gravity and physical exercise stimulate the digestive process and bowel movements. The medical world knows that sedentary, that is inactive, people, confined to a wheelchair or a bed, and astronauts have problems with their bowels.

Chronobiology

The moon is responsible for the cycle of seasons
and the stability of the axes of the earth.

Life on earth is linked to the cycles of the astronomical phenomena that manage days and nights, the lunar cycles, and the seasons. Our life adjusts accordingly during the different stages of our neurological, immune, and hormonal development, in relation to the rhythms of these phenomena.

Circadian rhythm

The circadian rhythm (Latin: *circa* = around and *dies* = day) is a cycle lasting approximately one day. For example, the sleep/waking cycle follows a circadian cycle of approximately 24.2 hours on our planet. This cycle is the most obvious of the circadian cycles. Science now shows that identifiable genes exist in our internal clock, and that the main area responsible for the slightly imperfect cycle of this clock is located in the suprachiasmatic nucleus of the hypothalamus.[13]

Several significant rhythms are associated with the sleep/waking cycle:

- the delta rhythm (frequency of 0.5 to 4 Hz), associated with deep sleep in an adult

- the theta rhythm (frequency of 4 to 8 Hz), associated with emotional stress and often present in brain diseases. It is associated with memory and learning and emotions

- the alpha rhythm (frequency of 8 to 12 Hz), associated with relaxation states in adults who are awake with their eyes closed (it is also associated with meditation)

- the beta rhythm (frequency of 14 to 60 Hz), associated with a relaxed individual focusing on a cognitive activity. More and more studies suggest that when the rhythm oscillates at a frequency of approximately 40 Hz (called the gamma rhythm), there is a distinct coherence in brain activity between different regions – a coherence that some describe as an extreme vigilance, an opening onto a new level of consciousness. This synchrony of brain neuron discharge would be the expression of the fuel of the spiritual experience in which everything becomes one.[14]

Deep sleep alternates with a rapid eye movement (REM) style of sleep. Dreams that we remember occur during this sleep phase. This sleep cycle is different for each of us. It also varies based on our life stages.

It is important to avoid being woken up when you are in a deep sleep. During deep sleep, referred to as 'slow', the parasympathetic system performs a repairing function by slowing down the cardiac and breathing rhythms, and by lowering the body temperature and blood pressure.

In the Western world generally we stopped having naps during the day and we go to bed only when night falls, when we don't force ourselves to stay awake until some ungodly hour, for all sorts of reasons. Barely a century ago, our ancestors slept approximately nine hours a night. With the advent of electricity, our night habits significantly changed: we sleep less and no longer take naps. It is due to social reasons and in an effort to be more productive (so to speak) that these refreshing naps have disappeared. When we try to bring them back, they are even met with flat-out disapproval, fuelled by prejudice and a lack of understanding.[15]

The *pineal body* or *epiphysis* is a gland that plays a major role in regulating the body's hormonal secretion cycles. It is not surprising that the hormone secreted by this gland, namely, melatonin, is directly influenced by lighting and is secreted at night, only *when it is dark*. These are therefore good reasons to wake up early and to go to bed at a reasonable time in an effort to help regulate hormonal production. Physiologically, we are not at all compatible with the illusion created by the invention of electricity and artificial lighting 24 hours a day ...

Patient and circadian cycle

After a good night's sleep, Sylvia, a woman in her forties, used to wake up at around 6:30 am, but was unable to fully wake up and be truly alert until almost 10:00 am. She would be tired in the late afternoon. To recover, she had to go to bed before 10:00 pm; otherwise she would have a second wind towards 11:00 pm and would be unable to fall asleep before 1:00 am. But when she went to bed at 1:00 am, she would wake up tired.

Many hormones are secreted according to a 24-hour cycle. In the 1960s research studies revealed in depressed people an abnormal circadian inhibition of the secretion of corticotrophin (ACTH).[16]

Cortisol is the key hormone stimulated by stress (see Chapter 13). The production of this hormone varies according to a predetermined pattern, within 24 hours. The highest levels are reached towards 8:00 am, followed by a sharp decline: a slight rise occurs at noon, and then the most dramatic drop of the day that ends at around 4:00 pm. There is a subsequent increase towards 6:00 pm, then a decrease until the brief upturn at 11:00 pm.[17] When the adrenal glands are exhausted, we lack cortisol when we wake up: it is not surprising that we are tired all day and more sensitive to changes in this hormone's daily cycle. That late afternoon fatigue is partly explained by a less significant secretion towards 4:00 pm. And the renewed energy just after bedtime goes hand in hand with the final peak of production in the day. Cortisol works in conjunction with insulin to maintain an adequate cellular level of glucose, based on the required energy demand. It is therefore important to coordinate the frequency and quality of the snacks consumed to be able to optimize energy levels at different points of the day.

Weekly cycle

The Sabbath has only existed for approximately 5000 years. It is a day of rest on which nothing that could be considered work is done: this day falls on Sunday for Christians, Saturday for Jews, and Friday for

Muslims. In Western society the weekend rest period has only existed for a few centuries. This concept is on its way to becoming a thing of the past since the arrival, in the late twentieth century, of stores open for business 24 hours a day, seven days a week. Working from home increases flexibility from family and time-management perspectives but, for some people with perfectionist tendencies, there is a risk of offsetting the balance of the 'work-rest-work-rest' cycle that then becomes 'work-rest-work-work-work-work-flu', etc.

Monthly rhythm – menstrual cycle

When you have no more energy to spend, you realize just how energy-draining menstruation is. It is clearly a time during which there is a significant energy demand: the need for energy to rebalance the human body's internal homeostasis is much greater. The hormone levels just before menstruation demand sustained work on the part of the endocrine system and the liver, which possibly physiologically justifies the drop in energy and the increase in symptoms in some women suffering from persistent fatigue. The loss of blood, especially when it is abundant, requires an increased contribution of iron. In his book *The Stress of Life*, Dr Hans Selye writes that premenstrual syndrome (PMS) is 'very similar to the deoxycorticosterone intoxication syndrome'.[18] He also adds that the Pakistan medical journal *Medicus*,[19] suggested in one of its editorials the terminology of *premenstrual stress* and described such a state as a derailment of the general adaptation syndrome.

Migraine headaches and oestrogen dominance

The so-called bilious migraines I was suffering from almost all coincided with my ovulation and with the day before my period started. After ovulation, there was a consistent increase in oestrogen level that would decline after my period. Just before ovulation, there was also a slight increase. The hormonal fluctuation is extremely taxing for the liver and energy-draining for the body–mind's homeostasis. When the menstrual cycle is anovulatory – that is, when progesterone is not produced by the corpus luteum – the stress level is even greater.

Oestrogens can cause the brain, as well as the breasts, to swell. These hormones can also deplete the magnesium reserves. In Chapter 5 we saw that a magnesium deficiency has a tightening effect on the muscles and arteries. The arteries thereby become more prone to spasms, a common cause of other types of headaches.[20] Dr Lee makes a connection between *oestrogen dominance* (excessive oestrogen that disrupts the hormone balance) and gallbladder disease (see Appendix 1). This may explain why persistent fatigue is more common and more easily identifiable in women.

Energy demand of female monthly cycle

Kate, Josie, Katarina and Lee-Ann are all women between 35 and 47 years old who noticed, when they used the Daily Energy Scale, that their energy level would drop considerably three to ten days before their period, based on their degree of overall exhaustion.

A note for men suffering from perszistent fatigue: if you are exhausted by family conflicts, it's obviously not related to your monthly hormonal cycle, but perhaps to that of your spouse...

Cycle of seasons

We know that among certain animals, hibernation is an annual physiological phenomenon. We also know that the mating season among animal species is seasonal, and is related to the more or less brief day/night cycles.[21] It has been noted in the hospital field that cerebrovascular accidents (CVA), or strokes, occur more frequently during the fall–winter and winter–spring transitions. In psychiatry we speak about *seasonal recurrence* as a factor to consider in people suffering from major depressive disorder. In an effort to explain seasonal depression, a vitamin D deficiency, resulting from a lack of exposure to the sun, has been suggested.

The rather chaotic, alarming, and accelerated pace of modern life shortens certain phases of one cycle at the detriment of another. We have the impression that we are dancing a waltz that continues to speed up, thereby destroying the harmony between the musicians, causing them to strike the wrong note. Finally, they have no choice but to stop playing due to disharmony, leading to cacophony, or imbalance.

Our ancestors followed the rhythm of the seasons. They would stay at home when snow paralysed the roads. There were no snow-blowers to clear the snow easily. They would be busy chopping wood to keep the fire burning and, before the advent of electricity, they would go to bed early. In the summer the heat would limit their activities. Today we have heating and air conditioning at work and in our cars. Basically, we produce without slowing down our pace.

Cycles of life

Many diseases are associated with the hormonal life cycle – especially immune-related diseases. During adolescence, in which hormone levels increase in both genders, minor problems arise: mood swings, migraines, and acne. After a pregnancy, sometimes conditions such as multiple sclerosis, Crohn's disease, rheumatoid arthritis, post-partum depression (which is, for many women, a set of symptoms, including hypothyroidism and nutritional deficiency, which contribute to a hormonal imbalance) arise or are exacerbated. Furthermore, for women, most diagnoses of depression occur in their thirties.

As a man approaches his forties, his testosterone levels decrease (there is a subsequent increase in the use of Viagra, because, after all, we live in an era of performance, whatever the cost) and the signs of overstress, obesity, and heart problems start to appear. Approaching fifty, prostate problems become more prevalent.

At menopause, hypothyroidism strikes many women. When an auto-immune reaction occurs, an inflammatory process is triggered in the targeted organ, creating an anti-inflammatory overload on the adrenal glands and, subsequently, on the entire endocrine system.

At retirement age, I noticed many cases of rheumatoid arthitis exacerbation in men who suddenly stopped working (mainly in men who had never had any interest other than their work). I recall a good number of clients suffering from heart failure, who had their first attack within the first six months of their retirement.

Changing habits to harmonize our own rhythms

In many belief systems, the source of the universe is a sound…a frequence. Therefore, the source of everything has a rhythm. Many believe that not being attuned to this rhythm creates disease.

We live in a world in which action is well regarded, as opposed to inactivity, which is not. However, after a person inhales, they naturally and passively exhale when they take control of their energizing breathing at the expense of energy-draining and inefficient breathing. The same thing happens with the heart: a contraction is followed by relaxation which fills up the heart with fresher blood on one side and collects the blood deprived of oxygen on the other side. Other cycles follow the same scenario: the body–mind needs sleep and rest periods after physical and intellectual work, the digestive system requires a period of calm when the person is eating in order to optimize its function, and so on. Human beings breathe in many ways. From a biorhythmic perspective, it is possible that *depression* is a very big exhalation after excessively frequent inhalations – exhalation, whose goal is to bring a life cycle back to its natural, innate rhythm.

Target at least one rhythm from the suggestions below that you want to regulate based on your own needs. Don't try all the exercises from one section. Be selective. Look for an exercise that seems easy to you and that you are interested in exploring. Approach it gradually. If you need assistance, have a professional guide you.[22]

Inhale–exhale

If you are very tense, it is possible that helping the breath to be more efficient might be a bit of a struggle at the beginning. Here are some little tricks to help you succeed at breathing calmly and efficiently without hyperventilating.

Lie on your stomach, on the floor, your head turned to the side, and bend the leg and arm of the same side for greater comfort (see Figure 7.1) Breathe through your nose without forcing. Observe how your abdomen and ribcage move, without trying to change anything. The advantage of this position is that you feel your belly push against the floor; it greatly helps to regulate breathing without voluntary control, while allowing the body to regulate itself on its own. This position is highly effective for people who have an inverted respiratory pattern. The position is also useful for observing the discomfort of mouth breathing as well as the possibility of sleep apnoea in some people.

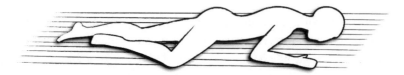

FIGURE 7.1 Breathing rhythm awareness position

I personally like to do singing exercises in the shower. Singing a long note to the sound of 'aaaaaaahhh' is enough to facilitate effortless breathing. After five sung exhalations, my breathing rhythm regulates itself on its own and I can focus on my activity. If you don't want to or cannot sing, do it in your head: it works just as well! Breathe in using the belly and pretend to sing a steady note until you have completely emptied your pulmonary 'ballast'. Wait until the next inhalation. It is possible that it will regulate the movements of your belly itself. It is possible that you will experience spasms in the diaphragm and that your emotions will come out. This is completely natural: blockages gradually clear up, easing tensions caught in the tissues of the organism. Let yourself go. If the moment isn't right for expressing your emotions, or if you don't have the energy required to handle them, return to the exercise later. Make sure you're always enjoying yourself.[23]

Alternating breathing is a type of breathing taken from *pranayama techniques* of yoga, that consists of breathing (inhaling–exhaling) through the left and then the right nostril for one breathing cycle. Similar techniques are part of Buddhist traditions and the Padovan method, which is more contemporary, is what I use with my patients. After an initial inhalation, you block the right nostril and exhale through the left side. The following inhalation will occur through the left nostril. Then you block this nostril to exhale out of the right side. Then you inhale through the right side, etc. This technique helps to improve the quality of the breathing of each side of the sinuses (avoid using this technique in the case of blocked nostrils as a result of a nasal infection, sinusitis, rhinitis). It has been said that alternating breathing is effective in balancing the two sides of the brain and in stimulating the nose hairs, thus the sense of smell. It would also have an effect on the stimulation of the melatonin hormone as discussed earlier.[24]

TAIJI AND QI GONG

In the PCPSP programme,[25] I teach breathing with visualization techniques designed to distribute and propagate moving *qi*. In addition to regulating breathing, this technique calms the turmoil of thought and activates coordination of bodily movement. Once the exercise is learned, it only takes a few minutes to regulate the ANS. It's an exercise that can be done during a break, at the office, just before a stressful meeting, or before starting your day. You can obtain more information on the technique from a Chinese martial arts association or from a qualified instructor.[26]

Systolic and diastolic contractions

If you do the previous breathing exercise lying on your stomach, you will easily be able to focus your attention on your cardiac rhythm once the breathing pattern regulates itself. Take some time to listen to the rhythm of your breath rather than that of your heart: the heart will harmonize with the calm introduced by the breathing. Note the systolic and diastolic contractions of your heart rhythm: the first one being stronger than the second one. Having one ear on the floor will amplify the sound of your cardiac resonance, and this will bring a feeling of well-being. Feel your pulse with your fingers on either side of your neck if you cannot feel it through your heart against the ribcage on the floor. By trying this conscious observation of your heartbeat a few times per week, you could become aware of your pulse at your fingertips. When you practise even more, you will feel your pulse through your entire body at rest at will.

When you listen to music, opt for ternary rhythms like waltzes, which have a tempo that harmonizes with your heart rate. Most people have a resting heart rate between 64 and 84 beats per minute. These rates are soothing, while fast binary rates counteract the natural heart rate. It is up to you to have your own experiences to optimize your energy level.

Peristalsis

In Chapter 5, you found several ways in which you could contribute to better consistency in your digestive rhythms. An environment conducive to calm and to being able to observe is necessary for effectively balancing the rhythms related to digestion, without having to be aware of making the effort to breathe, chew, swallow, and digest properly. Here are some additional points of advice to facilitate digestive consistency:

- Choose to prepare a meal or have a meal prepared that will simmer and smell good in your house long before it is time to eat. This will start the digestive process by triggering digestive secretions. You can also choose to eat in a place where you can smell freshly prepared ingredients.

- Eat foods with strong natural flavours that you enjoy: citrus fruits, fine herbs, tastes that you associate with energizing memories of your childhood (the healthy ones, of course), etc.

- Choose some foods that need to be chewed for a long time (meat, liver, raw or blanched vegetables and fruits) rather that softer foods.

- Avoid drinking excessively during meals.

Night and day

For some people, changing daytime habits is an approach that has greater success when they know why they are making such changes and when they have learned to love themselves enough to take care of themselves. To improve the circadian hormonal balance, I suggest that you make a few adjustments to your personal habits:[27]

1. Make sure you get outside every day to be in contact with sunlight. Even when it rains: it is beneficial to be exposed to outside light, rather than modern indoor lighting, for at least a short period.[28]

2. Go to bed earlier (not past 10:00 pm) to make reserves of the stress hormone, *cortisol*, secreted by the adrenal glands around 11:00 pm. Also, avoid staying up until 1:00 am. As often as possible, go to bed at the same time every night to reset and maintain your internal clock.

3. If you are in survival mode, go to bed at 9:00 pm or 8:00 pm, as needed! Even though you end up waking up at 4:00 am, eventually, it will rebalance itself.

4. Get the TV out of the bedroom in order to avoid watching it just before bedtime. This will prevent direct eye stimulation by the TV light that gives the wrong message to the hypothalamus-pituitary gland of the brain, sending the message that it is daytime when the body is supposed to be getting ready for nighttime. Moreover, this new habit will also be conducive to you finding some other pleasant, relaxing activities to engage in just before bedtime.

5. Sleep in complete darkness, closing your blinds totally, without using a nightlight or turning on the light during the night when going to the washroom. Turn the light screen of your clock away from your eyes and your body (you facilitate the production of hormones by the pineal gland which would stop until the next night if your body or eyes are in contact with light in the middle of the night).

6. If you work the night shift, and sleep during the day, simulate nighttime by making sure not to watch television just before going to bed, and sleep in total darkness. As needed, wear a mask like the ones distributed on aeroplanes.[29]

7. Make sure the temperature is not too warm at night: turn down the thermostat before going to bed. If you have cold feet, wear socks to maintain your internal homeostasis and to avoid being woken up by this discomfort.

8. Read something light that you find enjoyable. Avoid reading mystery or suspense novels, or even intellectually demanding books that stimulate your sympathetic hormonal system and your brain. The body–mind needs to be prepared for sleep and not woken up by the alarm of your fight or flight arsenal.

9. Just before turning out the lights, get into the conscious habit of taking a few breaths, or engage in a visualization exercise, guided by a CD or not, or do an exercise from Chapter 8 to regain awareness of your senses.

10. Listen to soft music that you enjoy.

11. Avoid eating or drinking just before going to bed: these activities disrupt sleep and the intake of liquid can lead to nighttime bathroom visits – especially if your adrenal glands are exhausted. However, if you suffer from hypoglycaemia and severe malabsorption, one hour before going to bed, have a snack that includes a complete carbohydrate and the same quantity of protein.

12. If your energy level is 40 per cent or less than your regular potential (see the Daily Energy Scale in Appendix 5), try to sleep until 9:00 am. As a result, you will bank the energy from the increase in cortisol produced between 8:00 and 9:00 am of the circadian secretion cycle of this hormone.

13. Avoid stimulants at the end of the evening: caffeine, nicotine, and moderate to intense athletic activity. For some, a coffee or a piece of chocolate at 3:00 pm is enough to prevent them from sleeping.

14. Avoid alcohol, which induces less restorative sleep. In addition to having an unfavourable impact on the control of glycaemia, alcohol requires additional effort from the liver, which doesn't help to optimize the energy level. It is also a diuretic that promotes mineral loss.

For your information, based on your individual needs (consult a qualified healthcare professional), taking vitamin supplements such as vitamin B complex in ampoule form, magnesium and certain other tinctures, can have a beneficial impact on the quality of your sleep. 5-hydroxytryptophan (5-HTP for people who frequent health food stores), a precursor of *melatonin* and *serotonin*, can also be used on a short-term basis, *under medical supervision.*

If you take sleep medication when you need it, be aware that certain drugs like benzodiazepines practically act like alcohol and the combination of the two creates a cumulative effect. In addition, over time, you have to increase the dose to feel the same effect that you felt in the beginning. Over and above the long-term effects alone, addiction could develop. Consult your doctor.

'On the seventh day, he rested...'
Here are some good reasons for you to rest one day a week or at least half a day a week:

1. Take some time for yourself, alone, to get acquainted with yourself.

2. Change your frame of mind by reading something light, constructive, hopeful and maybe related to personal growth and development.

3. Spend time with your family, and do not follow an agenda.

4. Stop running against the clock.

5. Give yourself the right to *not* be efficient.

6. Take some time to do an activity that pleases you, to cater to your own needs.

7. Get reacquainted with the present moment.

8. Do what you always wanted to do and what you would always put off until later.

9. Laugh out loud.

10. See an energizing show.

11. Write down some of your own good reasons.

By the light of the moon

Generally speaking, we all have our ups and downs during the month regarding appetite, libido, mood, and quality of sleep. We need to be attentive to these changes rather than forcing our body into performing beyond measure. This approach improves the quality of life. I don't know if the moon influences us, as folklore would have it, but it is not difficult to jot down in our agenda four weeks of seven days. Moreover, women (not taking hormonal birth control) tend to notice these changes more because of their cyclical hormonal production of 28 days. But this is rather rare in twenty-first century urban society.

Here are some suggestions regarding women's menstrual hormonal cycle to help reduce the energy demand on the body that is already taxing their body–mind just prior to ovulation and gradually increasing up to menstruation and, for some, during the first few days of their period:

1. Avoid vigorous exercise a few days prior to and during your period.

2. Avoid greasy food, devoid of nutritious elements, just before your period and at ovulation. You will subsequently avoid taxing your digestive track and your liver, which is too busy having to deal with temporarily increased demands of hormonal management.

3. Take appropriate food supplements as needed and according to your menstrual cycle.

4. Hormonal supplements are also an option for some women with a more severe hormonal imbalance. As I am not a doctor and even less a gynaeocologist, I advise that you read the book by Dr John Lee and consult his website.[30] Consulting a healthcare professional in this field is necessary, because a lot of contradictory information exists, particularly with regard to bio-identical and synthetic hormone supplements, which are often mistakenly interchanged. Each woman has her own specific needs.

From one season to the next

During the summer, quality local fruits and vegetables help us to satisfy our energy requirements. When local food and the sun are more limited, everyone has to decide for themselves if there is an individual need for food supplements according to their energy requirements and their level of stress. Because of the well-known lack of nutrients in the Western diet, based on scientific facts regarding the effects of refined foods and sugar, mass production, and soil depletion, it is becoming increasingly recommended by healthcare professionals to add certain kinds of supplements to a normally balanced diet.

If your energy level does not exceed 40 per cent, I strongly suggest that you stay inside on extremely cold days. Staying inside would prevent you having to deplete your energy resources that you require to rebuild your system, while maintaining your internal *homeostasis*. If you must go out, dress very warmly so as to avoid having to needlessly contend with the cold. Extreme heat, especially on humid days, will also have the effect of reducing your daily energy. If you must go out, bring a snack and water so you can stay hydrated, as required.

If your energy is higher, you might not instantly feel the effects of the interaction between your body and climatic extremes, but fatigue will catch up with you at the end of the day. Even athletes notice greater fatigue after engaging in athletic activity in extreme cold or extreme heat. If you are in an urban environment, be aware of the repercussions of climate on the quantity of smog in the air. Beware of air conditioning: my exhausted and mineral-depleted patients have almost instantaneous energy losses when they are exposed, even briefly, to this type of refreshment.

> *Climates, seasons, sounds, colours, light, darkness,*
> *the elements, aliments, noise, silence, motion, rest,*
> *all act on the animal machine, and consequently on the mind...*
>
> Jean-Jacques Rousseau

Reconnecting

It seems that some people suffering from persistent fatigue are disconnected from many of their own different types of breathing patterns: inhale–exhale, work–play, talking–listening... This leads to a hormonal derailment which can be seen as a metaphor for this disconnection with our environment in the five dimensions of our lives.

Have a good time reconnecting in your own way!

Chapter 8

Breaking Free by Rediscovering Your Body

Our body...our temple.

We are part of an environment that has an impact on each and every one of us. We can avoid certain situations, but it is not always possible to skirt around the stressor or stressors. What can we do if we find ourselves faced with an unavoidable energy-draining environment or situation? How can we modify our approach to decrease its effects on our body–mind?

For people suffering from *persistent fatigue*, the body's inner balance has clearly been disturbed, which explains how critical it is to gain a deeper understanding of the reasons for these drops in energy with which one must function during the various rhythms of a day, a week, a menstrual cycle, and during each season and year.

The journey back to a state of dynamic, healthy balance coincides with the body becoming reacquainted with its vital rhythms (discussed in Chapter 7). It is a sensory experience and this sensory information penetrates the nervous system through its base, the brainstem (see Chapter 12). It is here that lies the 'control centre' of the autonomous rhythms of the body–mind. Rhythm involves the notion of time and it is by rediscovering some of these rhythms in time that we are going to manage to regulate some of them that will have a beneficial effect on other rhythms and the entire psycho-neuro-immuno-endocrine (PNI) system and, accordingly, on every cell in the body. You are therefore now going to focus on your perception of time, which will have an impact on the energy you spend.

The concept of time

Do not dwell on the past,
do not dream of the future,
concentrate on the present moment.

Buddha

Dr Gary Kielhofner, occupational therapist, proposes a concept of time, based on the stages of life, which I will briefly explain here. A child perceives his life in terms of having a lot of time that lies ahead of him. His experiences are limited on account of an almost nonexistent past; he is eager to grow up, to become an adult. Although he is very involved in making daily new discoveries, his perception of time is more focused on the projection of himself in the future. An adult's perception of time is split between the experience acquired in the past and the future that lies ahead, all the while keeping in mind the daily responsibilities that weigh on the present. During the retirement years, the present can be appreciated through the perspective created by past experience. Memory and accumulated knowledge are factors that give the impression that a lifetime seems to be more behind us than before us.[1] This is what is shown in Figure 8.1.

In our modern and technological society, mankind has replaced the natural *clock time* or *chronological time* by the concept of *psychological time*.[2] Social and technological pressures constantly push us to project into the future to meet expectations in which performance; productivity and efficiency have reached excessive scales. We are adults with an acquired skewed perception of time that somewhat resembles the temporal perception of the childhood phase of life. But unlike the child, we disregard the present moment in order to constantly plan for the future. We do not live in the *here and now* and do not want to experience this present time, like that of early childhood, because we have adult responsibilities; we gluttonously consume each subsequent activity entered in our agenda. This process is energy-draining, even for a simple task that we do mechanically by rushing to be able to *survive* until the next activity in which we think about planning the third activity, and then the fourth, and so on, and so on... To live the modern way is to be in a perpetual state of urgency and our mammal's body–mind, although highly developed, was not designed for this type of perception of continual fight or this perpetual flight towards a later time. Apprehension, insecurity, annoyance, and fear take precedence, and these emotional states are often associated with this perception of time projected into the future. As a result, we even lose our sensory sharpness.

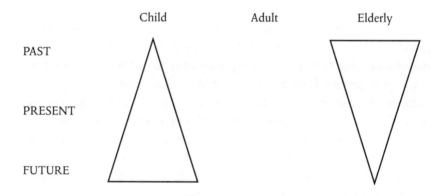

FIGURE 8.1 The temporal perception according to life stage

By disregarding the influences of the hyperconsumption and the overproduction of our society, some people, by their personalities and personal backgrounds, tend to focus more on *future psychological time*: they plan, control, and anticipate but do not pay attention to the activity they are performing here and now. They do not notice the beauty of the sunset when they are stuck on the motorway; they are too busy trying to slalom in bumper-to-bumper traffic hoping to reach their destination five minutes earlier. These people did not see the goals their child just scored because they were glued to their Blackberry, either talking with a friend or writing an e-mail to a client. The constant apprehension associated with this perception of time results in an unnecessary production of stress hormones and a loss of the natural rhythms of the work–rest cycle.

Psychologically, other people prefer to focus on the past. These people tend to live immersed in regret, guilt, shame, anger, sadness, and nostalgia. They dwell on the past, regardless of whether it is positive or negative, almost completely avoiding what the present has to offer. They feel guilty, play the victim, or always tell the same stories, good or bad, of the past, or blame the unmet needs of their childhood. All these behaviours disguise the present moment, whether it is pleasant or not. Too often, this illusion diminishes the production of neurotransmitters related to energizing emotions and increases the production of energy-draining stress hormones.

At the extreme end of the spectrum, there are people who lose themselves even further in the illusion. These people attach importance to the psychological time of the past and of the future and almost entirely avoid *being* in the present. Avoiding the present may mean that the here and now is uncomfortable or at least incomprehensible and anxiety-provoking. Figure 8.2 provides a visual way of looking at these three extremely distorted perceptions of time which have a major energy-draining impact on the body–mind. All these processes numb the info-energy harnessed by the senses, that is, it decreases our body awareness and, accordingly, upsets the sense of awareness of who we really are.

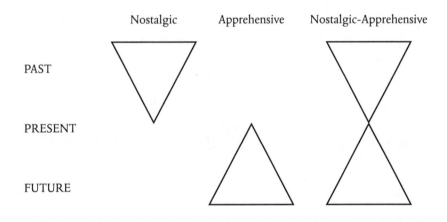

FIGURE 8.2 **Energy-draining perception of time**

In playful activities like dancing, painting, gardening, playing a musical instrument or engaging in a sport or martial art, what often unconsciously attracts us is the quest for the present moment: one even says 'losing the notion of time' of this moment. Knitting and crochet had the same effect for our grandmothers. Fishing and hunting for our fathers. The activity can stimulate this appreciation of the present moment and help us pay attention to this 'here and now' of space-time, through our senses. More and more people need to climb into racing cars or engage in extreme experiences to feel something that is accessible to everyone on a daily basis. For those who know how to go about this without accomplishing major feats or risking their life, engaging in extreme activities is not necessary.

The key point is summarized well by Eckhart Tolle: 'use the time-clock required to live in society but avoid psychological time, which exhausts us...'[3] as illustrated by Figure 8.3. To help us be more present, there's nothing like rediscovering breathing during activity and the info-energy,[4] which is transmitted to us by our senses. Observation of senses in the present is a highly effective way of changing our perception of reality and of distancing the conditioning filters that we have developed to interpret the information received. It's the return to an energizing and energy-saving way of life.

PAST

PRESENT

FUTURE

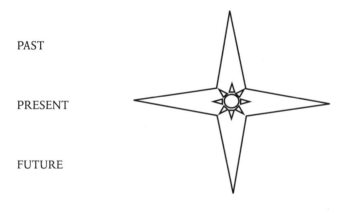

FIGURE 8.3 **Being in the present: taking into account the 'clock time'**

This technique is called *distraction* and is widely used in cognitive therapy to stop the draining ruminations of people's inner speech. Old-world wisdom leads me to think that this method is more than a simple method of *cognitive distraction*. Giving special weight to moments during the day in order to have a conscious experience of the present time has a considerable and favourable power on the biochemistry of the body–mind: this change in habit modifies the response of the internal messengers of info-energy. It is a powerful neuro-hormonal regulating tool of the body–mind.

Re-establishing the regulation of the autonomic nervous system

Scientists such as Dr Candace Pert have found that emotions and sensations are related in such a way to one another that they influence and modify each other.

Adrenaline and cortisol flow in abundance like the messengers of our body's response to stressors when we activate our sympathetic nervous system and our survival glands: the adrenal glands (see Chapter 13). We often add stimulants to them to go faster and to do more: caffeine, sugar, synthetic hormones, and drugs: illusions of panaceas that are increasingly widespread in all levels of society.

To regain control over who you are, to decrease apprehension when faced with the unpredictable and the new in daily life, to stop being constantly bulldozed by the illusion your ego has of being threatened and playing down the incessant ruminations in your head that are rendering your state of health even more fragile, this is what I propose...

It's a matter of being anchored in the activity in which you are engaged without being concerned about the incessant flow of thoughts; the issue is not to stop such thoughts, just to avoid lingering over them. Considering future schedules does not mean continually worrying about knowing whether you are going to satisfy them or not. Being present in the activity here and now does not mean forgetting the past, but rather applying your knowledge and past experiences to enhance the present in order to make the best possible decisions in the present time.

Often events throw us off and we lose all sense of meaning regarding our activities, our concerns, and even our life. Returning to the present moment allows us to rediscover, through our senses, who we are and what is important in itself. It allows us to clarify our relationship with our environment. For our life to have meaning, it is important to effectively use our senses...

In the 1970s Gestalt therapy explained how to be *here and now*. It is currently proposed that we let go of psychological time to more effectively use chronological time.[5] It is not so difficult to find our way because one thing remains constant: the importance of the present time.

Paying attention to your body's sensations, here and now, will help you to better respond rather than react. You will regain a certain control over your life and with a bit of experimenting, it will diminish the perception by the ego of threat or apprehension. All the channels of sensory information pass by the primitive brain located in the brainstem (see Chapter 12). At this level, several interactions form between the sensory nuclei of the cranial nerves and the rhythm control centres of the ANS. This is produced well before the info-energy arrives at the cerebral cortex. The very fact of anchoring you in your bodily sensations is a very powerful way of reducing stress and distress.

The following is a brief description of the phenomenon that acts on our body–mind:

Reducing tension by paying attention.

Exercise 8.1: Living in the moment, paying attention

In the exercise outlined in the physical Energy Balance Sheet (Chapter 3), you observed your way of functioning in relation to the ANS and its sympathetic and parasympathetic branches. First observe to what time perception you are referring during these same activities. For example…

Taking a shower in the morning

Are you living in the future 'subsequent' continuous tense?

- Do you plan your day while taking a shower?
- Do you think of what you are going to eat for breakfast?
- Do you listen to the noise the other family members are making to try to figure out what they are doing?

Are you living in the 'recomposed' past continuous tense?

- Do you ruminate about what happened at the office or with your spouse the day before?
- Do you attempt to relive the scenario of the past that you regret: an impatient word with the kids or work colleagues, a bad decision taken last week or last year, etc.?
- Do you continuously reminisce about the good old days, at a time when you did not have the daily worries you now face?

There are reasons to avoid the present moment, but for now let's focus on reinstating that moment. Once the observation has been made, try to find a way of being in the present during these activities. The idea behind these mindfulness exercises is to rediscover daily activities through your senses, almost as if you are doing them for the first time, through new eyes, with a clear ear, a subtle touch, a refined nose, alert taste buds, and a conscious presence with respect to your body (proprioceptive and vestibular) with regard to its accurate and energy-saving movements (kinaesthetic) in space. To be successful in this exercise, it is enough to observe the subject of your thoughts during these activities. You can even observe your resistance to doing this exercise. It is not a matter of judging, cataloguing, blaming, simply observing.

Use Table 8.1 to help you remember the sequence. Enter the anchoring activities that you use and ask yourself if you gave special weight to the *sympathetic* or *parasympathetic* system during the few minutes the exercise lasted. What conclusion do you draw? An increase or a decrease in energy after this activity? Enter your comments.

Let's summarize the exercise with a concrete example.

Taking a shower in the present moment

- *Breathing:* Take a few deep breaths, then observe the impact on your breathing. Just this gives you the opportunity to adapt to a less productive perspective of the activity.

- *Position in space:* Close your eyes and focus on the space occupied by your body in relation to the confined environment of the shower; focus on the information provided by your feet in contact with the floor of the shower stall; note the imprint of your feet on the floor. Notice how your shoulders may be fighting for no reason against gravity; feel the subtle sway of your body at each moment, correcting your posture to maintain your balance. Note the tremor of your eyelid if you are very tense.

- *Hearing:* Listen to the noise of the shower, of the water falling down on the floor, the friction of the soap on the facecloth…

- *Smell:* Keep your eyes closed to focus better on the smells: the subtle chlorine or metallic odour of the water, the soap, the shampoo, the shower gel, and your body.

- *Touch:* Keep your eyes closed or half closed a little longer and take a moment to feel the contact of your facecloth or shower gel on your skin, the contact of your hands washing your hair. Is it pleasant or uncomfortable? Is the water temperature pleasant? Observe without judging; the *emotional expense* of the value judgement causes you to waste energy.

- *Taste:* Do you taste the humidity in your mouth? Is it pleasant?

- *Sight:* Now open your eyes and look at the objects around you, the soap, the taps, the shapes, as if this were a new experience.

- *Position in space:* Keep your eyes closed and observe one more time the imprint of your feet on the floor, the sway of your body, and the quality of your breathing: are these the same sensations you felt at the beginning? If not, do you notice the difference? Are your eyelids trembling as much?

- *Breathing:* Observe your breathing and feel the difference.

During each of your activities, you will realize that your thoughts keep on taxing your nervous system like an old record that keeps playing incessantly: this phenomenon prevents your body–mind to balance itself. You are using a useless *cognitive energy expense* to accomplish this activity. It is as if you were making a tight fist all day long, regardless of whether you were reading, walking, or watching TV, without giving your muscles a chance to rest. You may suffer from cramps and an accumulation of acid in your muscles. Within a very short period of time your muscles' ability to efficiently contract may tremendously decrease. This is what happens to the nervous system when you do not allow it to restore itself: it gets all worked up, fills up with toxins, gets thrown off, and, finally, becomes exhausted. So find a way to return to the present. The return to conscious breathing brings you back to the present and decreases this energy expense.

In the beginning, you may notice more symptoms related to your *malaise*. It is not a matter of new symptoms, but only the consequence of greater self-awareness and the realization of what you have been avoiding, either consciously or unconsciously. It is no coincidence that you have been living somewhere other than in the present for a long time. Certain realizations will simply occur as you become more attentive to your body. Ultimately, there will be a favourable impact on this pain, this discomfort, this tension etched into the background. And on to this malaise that you have been handling for so long…

Qualitative changes will gradually occur. Begin by recognizing what is present. Do not struggle against information that your body–mind is sending you. Little by little, the resistance, then the malaise, will dissipate. But maybe not the first, second, or third time. Be patient. Be indulgent with yourself.

After having done this exercise in the daily activity of your choice, always the same activity, several days in a row, you will start to perceive yourself differently. You will view your environment with a new awareness: a cloud in the middle of downtown, budding blossoms in springtime, the moon and stars, despite the city lights, the smells of country vegetation. All this will thrill you as if you were being given glasses specially adapted to you. It is a wonderful thing, this present that starts to inhabit you. You get to like it.

TABLE 8.1 Daily anchor activity

WEEK...	MONDAY	TUESDAY	WEDNESDAY	THURSDAY	FRIDAY	SATURDAY	SUNDAY
Chosen activity							
S or P?							
Energy level							
Comments and impressions							
Imprint (before) Position in space Breathing							
Other senses Touch Smell Taste Hearing Sight							
Imprint (after) Position in space Breathing							

Legend: S = Sympathetic, P = Parasympathetic, ↑ = Energy increase, ↓ = Energy drop.

In the beginning, choose times of the day that are most likely to be conducive to completing this kind of exercise. For me, the shower is the ideal place because there is likely to be the least interruption possible. If you succeed in being present for two minutes of the activity that you are doing, this is a step in the right direction. Congratulations! Health breaks and repetitive and automatic activities (like walking, taking out the rubbish, doing the dishes, waiting in line at the bus stop, at the bank machine, etc.) are *special daily moments* in which it is easier to focus your attention on the information that is continuously grasped by your senses. Don't try to beat the clock; the activity you are doing is important, because it is allowing you to *be*. Go slowly. Be gentle and understanding with yourself. And the most difficult part is to refrain from trying to be productive, from having expectations. Experiencing this moment in space – here and the time – now 'without goal or benefit', just *being*. That's already enough in itself.

The bother of the daily routine wears on you, perhaps from the time you wake up. In this case, write what you have to do for the day once you get out of bed, or even the night before if you have the energy to do so. In this way, the whirlwind of planning will not leave you feeling overwhelmed.

The very fact of focusing your attention on the present moment will transform the way in which you do an activity. The focused attention will harmonize your speed of execution and will decrease the amount of energy required to accomplish this activity. The walking pace will adjust itself if the illness does not already force this pace to slow down. And the walking pace will in turn make breathing easier. The strength with which you close a door will be lighter and more effective. Movements will become more accurate over time. The volume and intensity of your voice will gradually modify itself, therefore saving you energy.

I am adding another activity here whose functions depend on a balanced ANS. We are referring to eating meals. It is very difficult to be present at meal times in a world that is incessantly communicating. It is also difficult to eat alone without being interrupted, unless you lock yourself in your office, isolate yourself in a corner, off to the side, in a restaurant, or unless you wait for the entire family to eat before you sit down at the table. In these three cases, you risk being perceived as antisocial.

For practical reasons, it may be difficult to remain alone for the duration of a meal. In this case, find ten minutes, at the time of a break, to calmly enjoy eating a piece of celery. Disconnect the interfaces: the radio, the television, the telephone, the computer…

Eating a piece of celery (or a piece of apple if you prefer!)

While sitting comfortably in a chair, back supported, take several deep breaths and close your eyes.

- *Breathing:* Empty your abdomen and breathe in a few times to re-establish your breathing pattern. Observe this pattern.

- *Position in space:* Feel how your feet are rooted on the ground that supports your weight. Picture the imprint of your buttocks on the chair, mentally observe the curve of your spine from the lumbar area to the neck, and notice the tension. Observe your jaw. Now, be mindful of the saliva in your mouth. Is your mouth dry or not?

- *Sight:* Open your eyes and take a piece of celery. Look at its length, its colour, its shape, as if you were doing this for the first time. Observe the details of the outside lines, the inner smooth surface and its cut or broken sides.

- *Touch:* Close your eyes again and explore the piece of celery with your fingers. Touch the different textures. Is the celery smooth or rough? Do you feel it is cool or cold, as you take it directly out of the refrigerator?

- *Smell:* Bring the food under your nose in order to smell it. Do you smell its freshness?

- *Hearing:* Open your eyes and bring the piece of food next to your ear and close your eyes again. Listen to the noise of the food being manipulated by your fingers.

- *Taste:* Now bring it to your lips. What do you feel? Is it warm or cold? Hard or soft? Smooth or uneven? Bite a tiny bit off the piece of celery and observe which teeth bit into it and on which side. Then bite a second time. What do you taste? How intense is this taste? How you would you describe it? Now chew until the little bit is totally ground. Noticed where you store the little pieces of food prior to swallowing. On your tongue? In front of the tongue on your lower jaw? On the side of your inner cheek? Now mindfully swallow and notice the sensation in your throat. Take a few more bites the same way to finish eating this piece of celery that has become a new food, triggering many sensations.

- *Position in space:* When you are finished, close your eyes and take the time to observe: the contact of your feet on the ground, the imprint of your body on the chair, the alignment of your spine and the position of your jaw.

- *Breathing:* Again, observe your breathing pattern. What has changed?

Once this exercise has been carried out for several consecutive days, find the time, at least once, to have a complete meal in this way. If you are successful, try it once a week, without music or noise from the radio.[6]

No interruptions! You will not at all miss the news, your work overload... Instead, you will recharge your batteries and become more effective and relaxed for the rest of the day.

Summary

It's only when we truly know and understand that we have a limited time
on earth – and
that we have no way of knowing when our time is up,
we will then begin to live each day to the fullest,
as if it was the only one we had.[7]

Dr Elisabeth Kübler-Ross

The important point to retain from this chapter is that you find a moment in each day to live a little more fully in the present moment. The unavoidable activities of daily life can be perceived as being anchors for reaching this end result.

Do at least one unavoidable activity per day to recharge your batteries while adopting a more conscious attitude. During the activity, review each of your senses, one at a time. Although the old habits will not disappear overnight, you will be surprised by the beneficial effect achieved in a very short time if you persevere.

The convincing data shows that the attention given to bodily sensations during exercises involving full static (meditation) and active (in movement) consciousness are highly beneficial for restoring the functions of the PNI super system. It is therefore not a waste of time... And according to Eckhart Tolle, there are other reasons for doing this type of self-rediscovery:

Presence is needed to become aware of the beauty,
majesty, the sacredness of nature.[8]

Chapter 9

Breaking Free from Perceived Illusions

If the doors of perception were cleansed
every thing would appear to man as it is, infinite.

William Blake

In Chapter 8 we explored the benefits resulting from paying attention to what goes on in our time-space, here and now. The very fact of being present, through our senses, in that precise instant, has favourable repercussions on the autonomic nervous system (ANS) and on the entire PNI system. Let's continue the exercise of understanding the information received by our senses and of perceiving this information through our body–mind. By favouring energizing, rather than energy-draining, approaches, this understanding will help us to find other tools that are useful in restoring our balance.

What is perception?

Perception is the ability to meaningfully interpret sensory information.[1] To do this, we require several components: our senses, which provide basic information based on their sensitivity threshold; the quality of cognitive functions that process information at the level of the cerebral cortex; our emotions, which put this information in a context according to our emotional baggage; and, of course, our personality, which is related to the image we have of ourselves. Perception is associated with the constant inner dialogue, which results from all of our conditioning, conscious or unconscious.

Making sense of our senses

Our sensory receptors constantly transmit information coming from our internal (visceral sensitivity) and external environments. The information can give rise to an immediate change in behaviour, through a reflex arc – just like when the doctor taps the tendon of your knee (a local response at the spinal cord level). This information is sent to the brain at various levels that will react unconsciously with more complex long-loop reflexes, or that, after having judged the information as being relevant, will consciously respond to the information. The information received can be used in various ways:

- Unconscious reflex arc in the spinal cord: The doctor taps on the tendon in my knee and my leg reacts with a muscular twitch.

- Unconscious subcortical reflex: I stumble on the edge of the sidewalk and my body adjusts to prevent from falling.

- 'Fight or flight' reaction of the primitive brain influenced by the limbic system: A wolf bounds before me in the woods. I'm scared. My pupils dilate, my heart starts racing. The blood withdraws from my digestive system to flow into the muscles of my limbs, which enables me to run at top speed, or to get ready to fight based on what my survival instinct dictates.

- Cortical response that influences the initial reaction, therefore with a conscious component. My brain identifies the animal: If it is in fact a predator, I persist in my fight or flight behaviour, however, if I detect that it is a harmless dog, my brain deactivates the initial survival arsenal and calms the inner stand-to.

- Cortical response that interferes with the immediate reaction: I take an excessively hot cup in my hands. I instantly want to drop it, but I take the time to place it on the table so as not to splash the person directly in front of me.

- Subsequent, conscious response: I noticed, in the morning, that there was no more milk in the fridge. I am going to get some before dinner.

- Excessively delayed response with conscious and unconscious aspects: I am on my fourth glass of wine and I am drunk; I stop drinking and ask if someone can give me a lift home.

We don't all react in the same way to a given stimulation, that is, everyone has a different tolerance threshold to a given stimulus. According to the occupational therapist Winnie Dunn, 'persons who have high neurological thresholds require a lot of sensory input for responding … have a low sensory processing registration and do not notice sensory events in daily life that others notice readily… [Others] are sensation seekers and enjoy sensory experiences.'[2] Furthermore, '[p]ersons who have low neurological thresholds, or sensory sensitivity, notice sensory stimuli quite readily and more sensory events in daily life than do others'.[3] It is as if these persons were receiving information at a higher Internet speed compared to the rest of the population: as a result, they receive more information in a shorter time span.

When we are subjected to stressors over an extended period of time, or when we are suffering from post-traumatic stress, we become hyper-alert on a sensory level, which tends to overstimulate our ANS – in other words, the accelerator pedal of the sympathetic system takes control of the parasympathetic system's brake pedal. Other factors exist that accentuate hypersensitivity. When we suffer from insomnia or when we work at night, the awakening impacts sensory alertness. Other conditions, such as the migraine's inflammatory process, make us intolerant to light and noise during a migraine episode. A pain associated with a physical trauma, which has endured for a long time, can also heighten this phenomenon.[4]

According to Aron, Highly Sensitive People (HSP) are 'born with a tendency to notice more in their environment and deeply reflect on everything before acting… They are also more easily overwhelmed by "high volumes" or large quantities of input arriving at once… Mainly, their brains process information more thoroughly. This processing is not just in the brain, however, since highly sensitive people, children or adults, have faster reflexes…are more affected by pain, medications, and stimulants; and have more reactive immune systems and more allergies. In a sense, their entire body is designed to detect and understand more precisely whatever comes in.'[5]

Emotional brain

According to research, we now have proof that emotions have an impact on our immune, endocrine and neurological systems. Once we acknowledge this, the medical paradigm for health and diseases is likely to broaden in order to treat a super psycho-neuro-immune system.

To better understand the emotional brain, it is a good idea to clarify a few terms. Emotion is considered a generally intense, affective reaction, manifesting itself through various changes, primarily neurovegetative. There is therefore an observable response of the body–mind due to the combined reaction of somatic activity (ANS) and mental activity associated with an emotion.

The limbic system is the part of the nervous system that is responsible for the emotional colour of experiences that are significant to us. In other words, emotions can be classified into two categories: energy-draining emotions related to fear, and energizing emotions related to pleasure. To be able to memorize this information, our nervous system associates it with one of two deep emotional colours. According to behaviourists, we learn only to win a reward or avoid a punishment. This is the root of learning and motivation. More specifically, it can be said that we learn only when information is perceived as being relevant to us.

For example, when we go to school, we tend to enjoy subjects that we find easier (positive reinforcement = pleasure) and avoid those that we find difficult (avoidance of negative reinforcement = less fear, no punishment). When a piece of information picked up by the senses is neutral, that is, when it is neither associated with pain/punishment (energy-draining effect) nor with pleasure (energizing effect), it is rarely imprinted in the memory.[6]

Pleasure or Reward Circuit: In order to maintain the body's homeostasis and survival of the species, humans seek to satisfy their desires: drinking, eating, reproducing… When we feel good, when we engage in an enjoyable activity or participate in an intense athletic activity, we release the 'antipain messengers' called *endorphins*. The action of endorphins increases the level of the dopamine messenger and enhances this messenger's action, resulting in a feeling of well-being.

To have a good understanding of the manner in which we behave, it is important to note that the prefrontal cortex is very rich in dopamine messengers, which is involved in controlling our irrational and impulsive behaviour. One of the consequences of the increased *dopamine* in the prefrontal cortex is sharper attention paid to the activity in which we are engaging.[7] The more successful you are in an activity, the more you secrete chemical neurotransmitters that maintain good cognitive performance and reinforce the sensation of well-being.

Pain or Punishment Circuit: With the help of functional magnetic resonance imaging (fMRI), researchers demonstrate that electric stimulation of the cerebral amygdala especially evokes *fear*, sometimes irritability, even anger. This *limbic system* structure is at the heart of this circuit. This is the circuit that is set in motion to avoid any threatening danger, and which gratifies us by the flight or favourable outcome of the fight. When we are in a state of fight or flight, we activate the sympathetic branch of the ANS, which discharges noradrenaline in response to stress. Visceral reactions are exposed in greater detail in Chapter 3.

Physical activity is medically recognized as an excellent way to reduce stress after a particularly demanding day, during which it was impossible to fight or flee. Physical activity reduces the harmful effects of stress.[8] Why? Because we all secrete these stress hormones to fight the threatening 'black bear', the 'big mammoth', or its everyday equivalent in traffic, at work, or at the supermarket. Unfortunately, we can neither fight nor flee when we are sitting in the driver's seat, in an office chair, or in line to pay at the supermarket. We remain overloaded with stress hormones – excessively overloaded, and this, over the long term, will potentially have a toxic effect on our brain's limbic system. In Chapter 1, you familiarized yourself with a list of cognitive and emotional symptoms associated with stress and persistent fatigue. These symptoms are associated with the prefrontal region of the brain in charge of emotions and learning.

In terms of survival, it has always been more important to remember threatening and energy-draining events rather than energizing events: our ancestors' mad race in the direction of a big rock to seek protection from the bear unable to climb was more beneficial for survival than the meal taking place next to that very rock. That is why, from a survival-of-the-species perspective, in most situations, an energy-draining memory takes precedence over an energizing memory.

Two cerebral hemispheres: we know that each cerebral hemisphere is specialized in its functions. In terms of expressing emotions, Dr Davidson and his colleagues demonstrated that the two hemispheres have asymmetrical emotional responses.[9] The left hemisphere is associated with energizing expressions of emotion (*pleasure*), while the right hemisphere is associated with energy-draining expressions (*fear*). Our emotional disposition is subjected to our temperament, and therefore possibly to our cerebral dominance.

Essentially, what motivates our behaviour with respect to the information received is not exclusively sensory. There is also our personality, the expectations associated with the context, the emotional state in which we find ourselves, the education we have received and our conditioning (i.e. the response loops programmed over time to deal with this type of information). These functions serve at the level of the limbic system. There are therefore conscious and unconscious (emotional memory) reasons behind this state that influence our perception and, consequently, our behaviour: 'I continue to excessively consume alcohol or be too hard on myself: this behaviour leads to self-destruction because I punish myself with an unconscious guilty feeling,' or rather, 'I want others to take care of me to satisfy an emotional need,' etc. The childhood conditioning that motivates us is more extensive than we think: 'I cannot stop eating because my mother always told me to finish everything on my plate rather than listen to my stomach.'

Cognitive skills

Cognition is all the mental functions that make up our thoughts. These mental functions are: attention, memory, and complex organization functions of information. Cognition is a process that leads to knowledge, an appreciation, intuition, an awareness of our environment and of what we are experiencing in this environment. It puts information in context. It is an important step in the perception and learning process. Each lobe of the two cerebral hemispheres, and of the cerebellum, processes information, according to its specialities. Magnetic resonance has shown us that a person's gender influences the processing of information much more than we believed when I was completing my university studies over 25 years ago.

To simplify things, I will say that the brain compares information with the entire *memory of sensations* – my databank of similar and dissimilar sensations (for example: the sensation of broken glass under foot: pain, heat-cold, light touch, pressure). The brain also compares the information with already acquired *knowledge* (processing of information), even if we haven't experienced this knowledge: 'I've been told that glass cuts like the blade of a knife.' It helps us to make informed choices: 'Broken glass cuts and causes pain. I'm going to put on my shoes and clean up the pieces before someone hurts themselves.' But if the sound or the sight of broken glass reminds us of the fear we felt during a dramatic event, like a car accident, for example (even if we don't consciously recall the episode), our perception and our reaction when faced with the broken glass will trigger a fight or flight reflex loop. It is as if there were two perception systems and the one that is unconsciously based on fear more often overrode the other. It is the *amygdaloid complex* of the *limbic system* playing a trick on the *neocortex.*

According to the overall model of understanding presented here, when our survival is being threatened, the limbic system takes precedence over the neocortex, the conscious, rational thinking headquarters. Without going into detail, we can conclude that the following information is important to retain: without interest or without a perception of the relevant aspects of the information received, there is no memory that is stored long-term, and: Fear takes precedence over pleasure for the survival of the species, but this trend can be modified.[10]

By discovering the relevance of the suggested exercises in this book, some of you will develop a greater interest in the exercises.

The ego: me, myself, and I

The I, or the ego, is the feature of our mind that helps us make decisions with respect to reward and punishment circuits. We initially understand that the ego is this 'I' that exercises choices between the primitive motives of the *id* and the demands of the authority of the *superego.* According to Freud, the ego makes its decisions for purposes of self-preservation. It makes decisions by controlling its motives on the one hand, and by complying with the rules that have been impressed upon it on the other hand.[11]

The ego is an image that we have of ourselves, which has been built, through our experience, within our family, our community, society, and the local and planetary environment. It is the product of our perceptions conditioned from the cradle, and it is developed with a sense of touch which puts a barrier between our bodies and the outside environment. It sets in before the age of two when a person discovers that 'I' is different from others. This 'I' depends on the angle of vision it adopts to draw pleasure or avoid punishment. It is a dynamic process that contributes to the feeling that one has of being an individual who is differentiated from others. This initial difference of the 'I' in its maturation process transforms over time, based on others, on the social good and on values less self-focused (egocentrism). When the ego achieves greater experience and maturity, it becomes more universal. It is then less defensive and considers 'us' (it includes itself in the decision-making process) more than 'I,' which is isolated from others.

In our society based on consumption and increasingly personalized products, individualism is currently much stronger than it was in the past. We live in a society that is hyper-centered on the individual, at the expense of the community, and this modern polarity toward the 'I' throws the relationships we have with the community off balance. Seligman even suggests that this excessive individualism would account for the depression epidemic seen in industrialized countries.[12] With this thrust of egocentrism, the meaning of life falls apart. In this context, we have a tendency to see the ego as an enemy, while it is a continuum that can vary in time and that has the potential to mature in an environment conducive to its development.

A 'solid' ego is an ego that has matured. It is humble, without false modesty and it knows its place in the world. This ego doesn't have an inordinate need for recognition from others and is not hypersensitive to rejection and disapproval. In this context, the power relationships between life instincts (the *id*) and the strict rules of the *superego* have less and less of a hold over it. They are subsumed, tempered: there is less repression, retention, extreme attitudes, exaggeration. This I, or ego, trusts in its abilities and accepts compliments with humility. It has good self-esteem. Maturity makes it calmer in its relationships with others. It agrees to live more in the present moment. Resistance gives way to resilience.

Little by little, the ego transforms itself by accommodating the collective 'us'. That allows it to have goals, to develop its sense of the common good, and to bring meaning to the life of the individual in relation to the community. As selfishness and egocentricity no longer take up as much space as before, the ego needs to *appear* less, and it therefore increasingly reflects what is essential for each one of us.

From which angle do you perceive?

What fascinates me the most in perception is each person's *angle of perception* when faced with the same situation.[13] Having supervised many employees, over the course of my practice, I would find it fascinating to see how a piece of information given at the same time to many people, by the hospital management, was perceived based on their needs, their sensitivities, and their personal interests. Whether it is the permanent or the temporary employee, the union representative or the executive, the professional or the technician, we had the impression that the individual was not in the same room as the others when the information had been given, or that he had not received the same letter as his colleagues with his pay cheque! Imagine for a moment the perceptual mess that results when fear and beliefs short-circuit our ability to reason. We can react to an employer, even to a spouse, just like we used to react to a parent when we were five years old. It happens daily, without detection. We can even react to a smell, a box used in a move, a car model, a uniform, in an unconscious and inappropriate way on an emotional level!

Having an angle of perception is necessary insofar as the brain receives too much information at once (just think about the distraction caused by roadside advertising when you are behind the wheel). The brain must select the information it receives and take only the information that is relevant based on the perception of its needs. However, too often, an awareness of our needs is submerged by automatic self-preservation thought loops.

It is important to understand that any perception of an activity or an event is influenced by beliefs and environmental conditioning that we carry around in our personal baggage.[14] According to the circuits we activate to perceive collected information, we use mental energy that could be energy-draining or energizing. By recognizing the perception we have of a daily activity, we realize the mental energy that we are expending. If we perceive it as being threatening or mandatory, it is possible that we are disconnected from our energy and have a feeling of uneasiness or *disharmony*. At this point the tension builds. In this context, we don't feel in control. For the time being, the ego is activated by using its self-protection automatic response mechanism. Influenced by the superego and primitive instincts, it accordingly plays a comfortable role for legitimizing its actions. In a given context, the emotions that it gives rise to are possibly completely unrelated to the activity in which we are engaged here and now. These emotions and behaviour have probably been necessary at a given time of our development and for the sake of our survival, but it is important to question their relevance in the current situation. These looped circuits that they have formed are perhaps no longer adequate here and now.

For example, if a man or a woman becomes very anxious and shouts at their spouse every time they arrive only five minutes late at a party, this reaction could possibly be an anxious reaction stemming from childhood, for having been severely and disproportionately punished for arriving late. This inordinate anxiety is in fact only an automatic reaction of self-protection interlocked by fear of punishment – a punishment that will not be endured but will be feared, because the punishment undergone during childhood stays in the memory.

Forcing yourself to artificially modify an emotion will not modify the perception that triggered this emotion, hence the importance of finding its underlying motivations and the thoughts that continue to contribute to such an emotion. When we realize that we can make changes in our habits for ourselves, we need *courage* to transform the reactive loops into reasonable responses that are better adapted to the situation at hand. By disregarding duty and the obligation of doing an activity (punishment circuit), we are changing our frame of reference. We are then allowing ourselves to accomplish this activity with interest (reward circuit), in accordance with our values, or we delegate the activity to someone else if it is unhealthy for us, or we change the type of activity, if possible. Cognitive behavioural therapy (CBT) brings us possible solutions to gradually transform our emotions and feelings based on our thoughts and our lines of thought. In other words, our emotions adjust when we change our perception or frame of reference. This approach triggers biochemical changes in the two above-described learning circuits (punishment and reward) and, possibly, in the configuration of the brain (neuroplasticity) of the reactive loops, but these changes have favourable repercussions on the PNI super-system and its self-healing mechanisms. All these processes result in an amplification of the feeling of well-being.

Exercise 9.1: Observation of the unconscious

Our ego is not our essence.

One of the best ways to bring the unconscious to our consciousness is to first observe our behaviour and our inner speech in each activity of everyday life. That is what you did in Chapter 3, in Exercises 2 and 3 related to the Energy Balance Sheet, taking notes on your emotional response and the perception you had of *duty* and *pleasure* with regard to each activity. By continuing this exploration you will certainly find solutions that will broaden your perspective or perception in the long run.

Return to the list of the four daily activities you have chosen. You can add other daily activities that are unavoidable and repetitive. Why? Because it is in performing small daily gestures that you are able to root yourself with who you really are. Since these daily gestures are necessary to achieve well-being in the household, they can rarely be avoided, hence the need to adjust our angle of view when we get caught up in the heat of daily activities. It is through doing these simple activities that conditioning may be easily observed. Rediscovering this inner observer teaches us to find out who we truly are beneath appearances, possession and performance. To be successful in this endeavour, use the guide in the box below every time you are on the defensive. Choose one activity for which you checked off 'Fear' and/or 'Duty'. Observe, and take note of your inner speech and its point of view regarding the feeling of obligation toward performing the chosen activity. If, during the time you performed the exercise in Chapter 3, you were not able to feel one or more specific emotions, it is possible that today, as you are conscious of your inner speech during this very activity, you may become conscious of the emotion you are feeling.[15]

Take the example of an activity that 'must' be done daily, for which I have included angles of perception of different individuals that can be modified according to the guide below.

The guide for energising thoughts

1. Look for a point of view in which dissatisfaction is perceived as *temporary*. In other words: try not to think in terms of *always* and *never*, in the absolute or in a way in which there is a *feeling of permanence*.

2. Be *specific* rather than *general* regarding what displeases you in the activity.

3. Avoid *self-demeaning judgements* and be more self-accepting. *Treat yourself with indulgence* in the same way you would treat your best friend.

4. Change your angle of perception of *lack of control* for a different one, allowing yourself to have control or at least a *feeling of realistic hope*.

5. *Focus on your senses and the present moment* in order to *avoid rumination* in your thinking related to an energy-draining event or situation unrelated to the activity you are currently doing.

Doing the dishes

Energy-draining inner speech:

- *Perception of permanence:* 'Why is it always me who gets stuck doing the dishes? It is not up to me to do this task because I have more important things to do.'

- *Overgeneralization:* 'I hate doing this chore because it is a lower-class job.' 'It's a woman's job, it's not for me.'

- *Self-demeaning judgement:* 'Doing such degrading tasks as these makes me a real idiot!'

- *Perception of a lack of control:* 'I hate this activity, water is bad for my nails and for my skin but I have no choice! Standing is not good for my back, for my health, for my varicose veins, etc.' 'I still have to do the dishes alone! My roommate doesn't realize I need help; he takes me for granted!'

- *Rumination:* 'Whether it's dishes or something else, my parents criticize everything I do. Nothing is good enough for them. They always find fault with what I do.' 'My mind is completely elsewhere when I'm doing the dishes; I go over in my mind everything that frustrated me today, yesterday, last weekend...'

Emotion: (a) frustration, (b) humiliation, (c) self-depreciation, (d) disgust or (e) injustice: 80%.

Now take a look at the activity from a more rational angle. Find a more energy-stimulating and less draining inner speech. Finally, *observe* the effect of this different inner speech on your emotional state. Do you feel the same emotion? If you do feel this emotion, do you feel it with the same intensity?

Energizing inner thoughts:

- *Perception of temporary:* 'If I don't *always* want to be stuck being the only one doing dishes, I will talk to my roommate and make a schedule so we will take turns, so I am not always the one getting angry alone in my head.'

- *Focus on the specific:* 'Whether it's a chore or not for a woman to do, I appreciate eating off clean dishes so it is important enough for me to do it.'

- *Be kind to yourself:* 'I am happy to be able to take 15 minutes and do something useful and automatic so I don't need to think.' 'The kids are doing their homework in the kitchen while I do the dishes: it's good to have the family all together after a long day apart from each other even if we're not all doing the same thing.'

- *Perception of control:* 'It's good to feel warm water on my skin and be able to relax while I listen to music.' 'I am going to wear gloves or cream to protect my skin.' 'I'm going to buy a footrest to lessen my back pain or sit on a stool.'

- *Focus on the five senses and the present moment:* Use the method shown in Chapter 8 to neutralize the thoughts buzzing around in your head and be conscious of the gestures and sensations associated with the current activity.

Emotion following changes to inner thinking: (a) frustration 10%, relief 30%, (b) humiliation, neutrality, 20%, (c) self-deprecation 5%, serenity 55%, (d) disgust 10%, contentment 30% or (e) injustice 10%, letting go 60%.

Energy effect: ↑ 'The fact that I have modified my inner speech stops the recurring draining thoughts in my head. The mental burden is reduced and I now have more energy when I do this chore.'

Do you feel a difference between the two types of inner speech? One conveys energy-draining thoughts that prevent pleasure from manifesting itself in your life. The other derives pleasure from carrying out an activity considered noble and necessary to any household. Imagine yourself in an activity in which you are very good, perform well, in which you have developed an expertise: just imagine the pleasure you could derive from an energizing inner speech! You don't become optimistic or less defeatist by repeating so-called 'positive' phrases that you don't believe. Instead, make sure you find a *rational* speech and not just nice phrases learned by heart that don't rhyme with anything.

To those who succeed at having an energizing inner speech and who have checked off *courage* and/or *pleasure* next to certain activities, I suggest that those individuals pay attention to the energizing inner speech that they sustain in this context. This speech will guide them to other energizing thoughts and beliefs and will shift their frame of reference – which will make the *fears* and *obligations* less gruelling.

If you did not quote *courage* or *pleasure* for at least one daily activity, look at the bright side: you have just realized something important and now have the tools to rectify the situation. For each of the activities you considered to be energy-draining on both emotional and mental levels (chores, burdens, duties, and obligations), identify the underlying thoughts of your speech. Write them on a notepad, especially the more recurrent and repetitive ones. By simply making the unconscious more conscious, you will open doors to change your frame of reference. Some activities might still remain heavy chores: accept this fact. However, many people will be able to change many daily moments to more pleasant ones and increasingly avoid the energy-draining habits. Do not forget that what you are looking for is an energy-saving mode but not necessarily in every activity: aim to achieve a balance between the input and output of energy. To the extent that the circuit of punishment prevails over the circuit of reward, I am making the assumption that over the long term, it is important to promote an energizing perception at more than 50 per cent to make a long-term successful change to the inner programming. Cerebral plasticity truly exists: it is possible to succeed. The recipe is simple: repeat, repeat, repeat…to create new habits.

Do not force yourself to change your emotional state, just accept it. Acceptance is one step in the healing process. It would be artificial and unhealthy to *force* yourself to change them. The thoughts underlying emotions are also a form of energy and if you do not manifest them in a certain way, they will certainly resurface otherwise. (Energy can neither be created nor destroyed. It can only be transformed.) All emotions have a purpose, so do not deny them! The self-protective reactions you have used in the past were very useful to you up until now to survive life's difficult challenges and events. Respect them, knowing that it is possible for you to adopt much healthier forms of adaptation.

Thanks to this exercise, you will discover that it is not necessary to force yourself to feel a different emotion than what you are presently feeling. Focus on a positive thought in which you do not truly believe will be even more energy-draining than accepting the emotion you are feeling here and now, regardless of what it is. It is really the observation and the realization of the content of the inner speech that will lead to a change in your feelings. The inner speech could modify your angle of view. Remember that changing your perspective will provide you with a whole new scale of colours on your palette of emotion. It is the pejorative illusion entertained by the inner speech that sponges on your energy savings. As such, look for an energizing inner speech in which you actually believe to stop the constant inner energy-draining refrain. In Chapter 11 we will address beliefs in greater depth.

Start with short, modest activities. The change in speech will change the frame of reference with regard to the context. This speech is contagious and will accordingly have repercussions in more complex activities in which a lot of unconscious behaviour occurs. Save the complex or more significant activities for the end. Take the time to savour your preparatory appetizers. Right here is the beginning of the end of your excessive usage of your mind's fuel. Several scientific studies show that we can change the frame of reference to shift, in daily life, from a pessimistic, energy-draining mode to an optimistic, energizing mode.[16]

Use Table 9.1 to write down your inner speech. Once you have successfully applied the energizing speech, if your energy seems to subjectively change based on your speech, make a note of it in the column *Energizing effect*. Draw an arrow upwards (↑) if such is the case, an arrow downwards (↓) if you feel worse, or a hyphen (-) if there is no change. It is possible that you didn't find an energizing speech to replacing the incessant, excessive, self-critical refrain. This means that you haven't finished your research. It's only a beginning. To finish the work, use the five components in the guide. Professional assistance could help if you are at an impasse or if you find yourself stumbling over using intangible obstacles or other defence mechanisms that were once useful to you, but that only prevent you from moving forward today.

The following are other examples of the daily activity exercise.

Taking care of a sick child

Emotion: powerlessness 90%, impatience 95%.

Energy-draining inner speech:

- *Perception of lack of control:* 'But what made him not listen to me and refuse to dress warmly. It's his fault if the flu infects our house. It screws up my routine. He's going to keep me up all night with his fever and his cough and I have a conference to give this weekend!'

Energizing inner speech:

- *Perception of control:* 'Another challenging flu to cure. We're going to take out the honey so at least the flu tastes good. We're going to aerate the house so we don't all catch it. I'm going to ask his grandmother to stay with him tomorrow night so I can prepare my conference. I will be in a better mood for having taken care of things if I finish my work.'

Emotion: powerlessness 15%, impatience 10%, relief 50%.

Energy effect: ↑.

Emergency at the office: prepare a document for a client at all costs

Emotion: disdain 95%, anxiety 80%.

Energy-draining inner speech:

- *Rumination:* 'Another unreasonable client who wants everything right away and who feels he's God.'

- *Self-demeaning judgement:* 'What's more, if I don't do the work pronto, he's going to think I'm incompetent and I'll lose him as a client.'

Energizing inner speech:

- *Focus on the present moment:* 'I take a deep breath and calm down to be able to deal with this emergency efficiently and stay in control of the situation and comfortable with myself.'

- *Be kind to yourself:* 'I provide good service without jeopardizing my health and perhaps the client will appreciate my efficiency and will respect me because I also set limits. If not, at least I will not have killed myself performing the task and I will maintain my health and my dignity.'

Emotion: disdain 15%, anxiety 25%.

Energy effect: uncertain.

TABLE 9.1 Observation of the conditioned inner speech

ACTIVITIES	ENERGY-DRAINING INNER SPEECH	EMOTION (%)	ENERGIZING RATIONAL INNER SPEECH	EMOTION (%)	ENERGIZING EFFECT (←→)

If you momentarily feel more tense doing this exercise, return to the simple conscious breathing. In the following chapters, we will examine other ways of dealing with these activities/situations loaded with emotions and tied to a memory of past experiences, to unconscious behaviour, and to old persistent beliefs. Healing is a process. Replacing old reflex loops with new conditioned healthier responses takes time.

If you want to fully tackle the inner speech and find other examples, I suggest that you read the work by Dr David Burns.[17] I know many psychologists and occupational therapists who use this type of method with their patients and who achieve very good results. Evidence demonstrates that cognitive behavioural therapy is an effective method for people suffering from persistent fatigue (with various diagnoses).

Chapter 10

Breaking Free by Taking Charge of Ourselves

Taking care of oneself before others is not selfishness. Taking care of others without taking care of our basic needs means going directly to energy bankruptcy that leads to illness.

The notion of respect seems pretty shaky in the society in which we live. Dictionaries tell us that 'respect is to regard with honour…to take care of…' Therefore, it means to regard ourselves with honour as well as others and the environment. In other words, it means to take care of ourselves, others, and the environment. Taking care of ourselves has nothing to do with being selfish; it is showing respect towards ourselves, that is, also accepting who we truly are and taking our own responsibility as adults in society. The obstacle is often related to 'knowing' who we truly and deeply are, because we are not what we do, nor what we possess nor what we think and even less so with whom we associate. We are also not the culmination of our previous conditioning and beliefs that were instilled in us when we were younger. Once we get to know a little more about who we truly are, it is possible to change our way of being with ourselves and with others. The better we know ourselves, the easier it is to position ourselves based on what pleases and satisfies us. We are then better able to assert ourselves in this context. Many people suffering from *persistent fatigue* do not have this recognition in one form or another. It is therefore imperative to first know ourselves before *recognizing* ourselves or being able to go ahead and enjoy recognition or, on a more basic level, others' appreciation of us… To once again learn to know ourselves, we must first understand that it is easy to 'confuse ourselves' with the demands of the inner critic, who communicates the conditioning and beliefs we have acquired over time. It is easy to confuse ourselves with desires or pseudo needs, which also stem from our conditioning. The ego is simply a perception of *ourselves*, a product of our cognitive process; if it is immature, it will remain 'selfish', 'self-centered', and this tendency will reduce our choices of behaviour when faced with daily life situations. Let's learn to recognize certain mental traps in order to discover who we really are beyond this hard shell, these multiple masks, these protective layers of onion that 'drain' a large part of the energy of the socio-cultural aspect of who we are.

The maturation process

Physiologically, we grow according to our growth curve. With regard to emotional and social maturity, and the growing responsibilities to be assumed as we age, we learn based on our individual abilities and on how we have observed our community: parents, teachers, friends, etc. From a cultural perspective, our perception is shaped by the media to which we are exposed and by the behaviour of political, artistic and scientific personalities to which we are drawn. Our cultural lineage is closely linked to the community in which we were immersed in our childhood, to the religious environment or lack thereof of the nuclear and extended family, and to Quebec's almost socialist and collective culture (I can only speak for my part of the world) embedded with capitalistic and North American individualistic culture. Everything is melted in a blurred, Judeo-Christian environment, which is beginning to open up, but which sometimes gets lost amidst other cultures.

First start by observing how you behave during your activities – those that you do for yourself and those that you do for others. It's through being more aware that you will be able to adjust your approach as needed with respect to many situations or activities in daily life. As a result, you will make more enlightened choices.

Self-protective automatic reactions

Our relationship with our*selves* and *others* is often at the core of daily energy-draining habits. Without being conscious of it, you may be attracted to people or groups of people who reinforce your conditioned perception of what you believe is – a perception in the spectrum of total lack of self-esteem to an exaggerated unrealistic, inflated self-esteem. This consequently drains your energy. The more limited self-awareness is during interactions with others, the greater the *social burden* in terms of energy management.

On a temporary basis, and according to circumstances, you can choose to position yourself in relation to others rather than in relation to who you really are. It is important to question that choice and the motivations underlying that choice. This way, you can decide if this behaviour towards others and towards yourself that you have learned continues to be relevant in your present situation as an adult.

We play different roles according to circumstances; roles we have learned through previous conditioning and that are now imprinted as reflex loops in our brains. Most of the self-preservation reactions are related to the relationships we maintain with *ourselves* and with others. Table 10.1 provides several examples of recurring patterns related to various mental self-protective reactions.[1]

TABLE 10.1 Recurring patterns related to self-protective reactions

POINT OF VIEW	COULD LEAD TO...	SELF-PROTECTIVE AUTOMATIC REACTIONS
The need to raise your self-esteem	*could lead to...*	moral judgement
Feeling threatened	*could lead to...*	attacking as self-defence
The need for approval	*could lead to...*	forgetting your own needs to assert yourself or tending to conform excessively to others
The need to be acknowledged	*could lead to...*	performing excessively
The fear of being judged	*could lead to...*	blaming others or becoming cynical
The need for self-esteem	*could lead to...*	diminishing others to enhance your own image
The need for a certain degree of control	*could lead to...*	guessing other people's thoughts
The need to be accepted	*could lead to...*	justifying yourself by being different (ethnic background or other)
The fear of being rejected	*could lead to...*	inertia, procrastination or stagnation

While our body continues to grow and age, our emotions are confronted with various circumstances, causing us to react. Such reactions occur when we find ourselves in the presence of certain people or groups of people who remind us of relational discomfort in our past, based on automatic childhood reactions. The power of the unconscious too often plays tricks on us and puts us in a situation of self-protection. The challenge here is to adopt a broader point of view to be better able to address the situation. The goal is to *go from an automatic mode to a thought-out action.* When we reflect, we shine a headlight on our own thought to clarify it.

There are more self-protective mechanisms acquired over time than there are examples. These are complex reflex loops that become *habit* and that we are not necessarily conscious we are using. Sometimes it is preferable to keep them as is, either because they are adequate, or because we do not have the professional support required to be guided to other more adequate self-protective automatic mechanisms, especially when we are faced with a particularly disturbing event from the past: an assault, a rape, a serious accident, an emotional shock, or a major disappointment. When we too often revert to our prior learning loop, we risk preventing ourselves from growing emotionally. These are 'reactive' and therefore energy-draining mechanisms. Like those in Table 10.1, they use the *punishment circuit* described in the previous chapter.

It is important to remain honest and respectful towards yourself, even if it is not always easy. To achieve this different way of looking at yourself, you may need a friend or a therapist to observe your behaviour. Outside assistance could help you to shake off your old obsolete reflexes and to maintain the healthy automatic reactions that enable you to sustain your emotional balance. It is important to progress at your own pace. In so doing, humour is considered one of the best automatic self-protection reactions. It incites us to be humble, and connected with those with whom we are laughing. Didn't Oscar Wilde say that 'life is too important to be taken seriously'? In Table 10.2, you will find other choices of behaviours that are more in line with self-satisfaction than with self-protection, without succumbing to selfishness or self-centredness. They further stimulate the *reward circuit* (see Chapter 9).

TABLE 10.2 Patterns related to self-satisfaction reactions

POINT OF VIEW	COULD LEAD TO...	SELF-SATISFYING RESPONSES *REWARD CIRCUIT*
The need for a sense of belonging	*could lead to...*	bonding humour
The need for self-satisfaction	*could lead to...*	altruism
The need for self-assertiveness	*could lead to...*	accepting our own limitations
The need for interpersonal relationships (togetherness)	*could lead to...*	sharing with others
The need for recognition	*could lead to...*	work well done
The need for self-satisfaction	*could lead to...*	generosity, giving of ourselves

What role do you play?

Memetics makes us play roles. If we change the memes that no longer suit us, we can break free from previous conditioning.

Self-protective automatic reactions are related to the conscious and unconscious roles we personify with ourselves and with others. Every automatic reaction makes us play a role according to the activity we carry out and based on the people present. Even when we are calmly washing the dishes alone, we sometimes play a role that we could identify only when listening to the reflex loop of our inner voice. This is what you did, in part, in the previous chapter.

What is important in this exercise is to realize that you are playing a role; observe this game, and become a little more conscious of what is going on. To illustrate, here is a non-exhaustive list of roles frequently discussed and observed in therapy:

- The *disenchanted cynic* in his vision of the world tries not to feel his deepest pain. Moreover, his defeatist perspective justifies that nothing can be changed, so what's the use?

- The *diplomat* makes sure that everybody feels comfortable in his presence but nobody really knows what he is thinking or who he really is.

- The *jester* is the comedian we really do not know under the steady flow of jokes.

- The *indecisive wishy-washy individual* changes opinions according to the people present and from one situation to another.

- The *warrior* fights for a cause, for his family and friends but will only fight for himself through the needs of others.

- The *indifferent one* removes and excludes himself from others to avoid getting hurt.

- The *independent one* never asks anything of anyone because he believes he can do it all, especially considering that he perceives asking for something as a weak character trait. What would happen to his *ego* if he asked for something and was refused? And if someone offered him help, how would he react?

- The *narcissist*, who admires himself, finds himself more competent than people around him, is self-centred, and is incapable of seeing anyone else's point of view.

- The *judge* is above everyone, and positions himself so as not to be affected by others' judgement. However, the criticism used towards others does not compare to the inner criticism that manipulates his *ego*.

- The *martyr* could give up everything, even his health for his peers or his work, his art…in order to gain a certain prestige for his excessively feverish ego.

- The *'botcher'* unconsciously settles for having less success than he is worth: he arrives late at his meetings, forgets a major deadline at work, finds jobs excessively beneath his ability and talents: this way he does not have to confront the change in his self-image and the glances of potential criticism from the outside.

- The *sceptic* takes the position of doubt only to doubt; as a result, he avoids taking a stance so as to avoid risking making a mistake or even being right!

- The *follower* hands over his life choices to a group (union, governmental, political, religious, ethnic, of common interests) because he does not know who he truly is and may not have received the tools to determine who he truly is.

- The *victim*, who feels stuck, deprived, never responsible for what is happening to him and whose purpose in life is determined by how other people regard his situation as a victim.

Let's stop here. To complete this list of roles, just delve into your traditional (religious and mythological writings) or contemporary (science-fiction films, tarot cards, video games) heritage and into your social sub-groups.

Start by not holding any grudge towards yourself.

Gotthold Ephraïm Lessing

Exercise 10.1: My self-protective system

The following exercise invites you to explore the old automatic reactions associated with the roles you accordingly play, and to evaluate their favourable (or unfavourable) effects on your energy level. Return to the exercise proposed by the Energy Balance Sheet. For each of the activities beside which you checked off *others*, write down your inner thoughts, and then try to find the self-protective automatic reaction that you used during that activity. You can also identify the role you play or, if you prefer, the position or the point of view that incites your mental side to defend itself. If you cannot clearly identify this role, write down your tendency by asking yourself the following questions: Do I tend to be demanding, aggressive, passive, indifferent, or passively aggressive towards others or myself when I play a role or when I use an automatic reaction to defend myself? Or do I truly assert my *self* in my behaviour and in my thoughts? Then, attentively examine the activity that you are carrying out. Awareness is the first step towards using more rational responses of self-affirmation and self-satisfaction. Ask yourself if this new perspective results in *comfort* or *discomfort*? The advice of an experienced therapist could help you if you feel a certain blockage or tendency to avoid during this exercise. Take the time to verify whether this *attentive observation* subjectively gives you an *energy intake* or not, and make a note of it. Do not judge yourself. The judge is the inner critic who creates a distorted perception. Instead, observe the sensation of *comfort* and the *energizing effect* as being the right indications to guide you. Use Table 10.3 as a clearing tool and add your comments.

To avoid redundancy, check whether the activities that are energy-draining on emotional and cognitive levels in the Energy Balance Sheet are partially the same as those next to which you had checked off *other* on a sociocultural level. If some are energy-draining, go back to Table 9.1 in which a part of the exercise has already been done. Simply identify a *self-protective automatic reaction* or a *role* to dispose of other knowledge and personal growth tools. Once again, you can take this step with repetitive daily activities to discover a wealth of information on the roles your ego plays and on self-protective automatic reactions.

Here is an example from everyday life.

Meal preparation

- *Inner speech:* 'I do not need help to make a meal even though I am sick and flat on my back. I should be able to manage by myself! I will reheat a frozen dinner!'

- *Self-protective automatic reaction:* Unrealistic expectations towards my*self*.

- *Role played:* The independent individual. Aggressive style towards my*self*.

- *Attentive observation:* Why not ask for help? The worst that can happen is you get 'no' for an answer. If I am told 'no', it does not remove anything from what I am worthy of as a human being and at least I will have learned to try to get help; and if I am told 'yes', I might even get enough rest to regain some energy and I will most likely eat a more nutritious meal to get better faster.

- *Comfort or discomfort:* Comfort.

Energy effect: ↑.

TABLE 10.3 Self-protective automatic reactions

ACTIVITIES	INNER SPEECH	SELF-PROTECTIVE AUTOMATIC REACTION	ROLE PLAYED	ATTENTIVE OBSERVATION	COMFORT/ DISCOMFORT	ENERGIZING EFFECT (↑↓)

Summary

Knowledge with conscience brings responsibility.[2]

Rachel Thibeault, occupational therapist

The first step to coming to terms with ourselves is knowing who we are and identifying what we need. Once we get to know who we are and who we are not, we gain more tools to be able to respect this precious being we have discovered – and its limits. Putting our own needs into perspective paradoxically brings us closer to *others*: it becomes easier to say 'no' to a tyrannical ego and to say 'no' to others so as to respect our own needs and limits, because we have finally taken the time to familiarize ourselves with our true needs and limits as opposed to what has been imposed on us. Coming to terms with ourselves also means saying 'yes' to activities that we enjoy without feeling guilty. It means saying 'yes' to the opportunities which do us good and 'yes' when facing the inescapable and necessary activities of everyday life without suffering through them, but by using our creativity to tame them and harvest our well-being. It is saying 'yes' to others in an energizing way rather than in an energy-draining way. This is how we can find and foster a better balance between energy-spending and energy-saving. Learning to face the challenges of everyday life enables us to avoid the mortgage of a persistent lack of energy and leads to better well-being across all activities, even the inescapable and repetitive chores of daily life.

Indirectly, when we adopt new patterns of protection or, better yet, when we perceive that we do not need to defend ourselves because doing so is not always necessary, we distance energy-draining people who feed off our more restrictive angle of view. The change in our manner of being is enough to trigger a rupture with unhealthy relationships or, rather, these people will strive to avoid us, or we will decide to create a distance between them and ourselves, and even to put an end to these excessively energy-draining relationships. Meeting new people with whom we can build energizing links will happen at the same time. We will also influence several people from among our peers, who will become less energy-draining where we are concerned, and also for themselves.

Chapter 11

Breaking Free through Conscious Interconnectedness

Mankind is part of the universe, not only its observer.

Illness limits us in our activities. The downtime it imposes often creates an opportunity in which we question what the activities mean in terms of certain values, which are also undergoing a transformation. Many ill people seek to find a meaning behind their illness. If the situation persists, they ask themselves about what their life means and about their goals based on their new image of themselves, their abilities, and their limitations. Activities that were once meaningful could seem ridiculous, while others, which didn't seem very important in the past, are now high on the daily priority list.

It is not the role of the occupational therapist to be a spiritual advisor in this context of personal questioning, but he is professionally compelled to guide patients so they may find meaning in their daily activities. He helps people reintegrate some of their previous occupations. He acts as a catalyst to make them discover new activities that are better adapted to their new realities. Furthermore, he can lead them to favour therapeutic activities that are meaningful to them – which will motivate them throughout their rehabilitation process towards a state of well-being. It's in this therapeutic perspective of activity that we will be addressing the theme of spirituality. Let's first start by defining this often vague term, which comes in so many flavours, and try to understand it in the context pertaining to our reality at hand.

Words like *respiration*, *inspiration*, *inhalation*, and *exhalation* share a common Latin root with the word *spiritual – spiritus*, which means 'breath'. Breathing implies a relationship with what lies outside of ourselves to which we are connected, consciously or not. Inhalation can be seen as the fact of agreeing to receive from the outside environment, and exhalation as a way of contributing to that environment. You will be able to approach the exercises in this chapter in such a way that reflects the nature of this relationship. They will give you the possibility of clarifying your priorities and choosing, in a more conscious manner, values you truly want to embrace. You will also have the opportunity to align your actions with your deep convictions. Having a better understanding of the values with which you truly identify will help you to see more clearly what it is that motivates you during your interactions with the people around you and with your environment.

Clarify

Although this chapter is the last one in the 'breaking free' section, it is the first one in which the opening and deep healing from inside to outside occur. For many, it is the beginning of the big overhaul intended to repair the dis-order lying at the source of the *dis-ease* that appears before the *disease*. People who have been struck by a violent accident or by a sudden illness experience *uneasiness* that possibly appeared after the initial problem. The *dis-ease* involves feeling disconnected from others and from the universe, and involves maintaining this feeling of isolation. It also involves an inability to detect meaning in the apparent disorder that surrounds us. By clarifying your relationship with the universe and by discovering who you truly are in this universe (which forms a whole), you will discover what is essential for yourself, in other words, what is, for you, a source of wisdom, beauty, creativity, and thus vital energy or personal power.[1] Positioning ourselves in a deliberate manner with respect to the meaning in our life synchronizes our actions with our deep values. Insofar as it defuses the effects of stress, this refinement of the body–mind harmony accentuates our feeling of *power* and ensures an optimal functioning of the PNI system.

Our overproductive and overconsuming society has conditioned us to *force*, to *perform*, to *own*, and to *appear* rather than to *be*. According to Dr Serge Mongeau, 'today the main social value is to…work, even if this work is useless or harmful, even if it is a task that is absolutely not suited to the person who is assigned to it'.[2] People lose themselves in work.

For many human beings conditioned by our modern society, life is divided 'between a work/leisure relationship in which the sole purpose of the second item is to relieve the first'.[3] People who work in the helping professions are the most affected. Astonishingly, however, this phenomenon is currently on the rise among blue-collar workers.[4] The social costs related to absenteeism are currently estimated at close to 20 billion dollars.[5] Fletcher believes that it is essential to maintain a 50/50 relationship between work and personal life, but this alone is not enough to achieve balance.[6] What makes us overconsume and be excessively productive is often the uneasiness derived from our conditioning and from our unrealistic beliefs in all aspects of our life.

In research related to work–life balance, 'life and living are generally seen as separate from working'.[7] In the daily work–life balance of activities, the meaning and purpose of these activities (occupations), their idiosyncratic nature, and their centrality to life are missing.[8] From an occupational therapy perspective, work is an activity integrated into the combined whole of all human occupations, and the more meaningful occupations there are, the greater the feeling of well-being, power, and vitality. An activity is deprived when what we do has no meaning or value for us.

On a physiological level, this disconnection results, among things, in increased stress hormones, increased inflammatory response, and a weakened immune system. We all need to feel that we are contributing to the well-being of society, that we are related, not 'disconnected,' from society. The individual who does not feel his contribution to the community perceives himself as being isolated, apart from society. He tends to 'push' to obtain things that only partially satisfy him. The other choice, for some, involves withdrawing into a passive state by avoiding making decisions related to their own lives. Many individuals find their own way of not 'feeling' their body–mind. In the case in which they are useful to the community, but are not aware of it – since their perception is biased by energy-draining, abusive conditioning – they have the impression that what they do is disconnected. But disconnected from what? From what they feel (on sensory and emotional levels), from what they think (on an intellectual level), from what they share (on a sociocultural level) and from what they believe (on a spiritual level), hence, from their vital energy. And their uneasiness can grow and imprison them in today's trap of *powerlessness*.

Beliefs and conditioning

From the psychiatrist David R. Hawkins to the biologist
Dr Bruce Lipton, it is now understood that our belief
system changes our body and influences our genetics.

Our beliefs are our thoughts' main source of conditioning. It is our beliefs that impose an angle of view upon us that leads us to observe and to understand in one way over another. Our entire personal upbringing forms the foundation of those beliefs, whether they are true or false. We think and act influenced, consciously and unconsciously, by the values conveyed by the place where we were born, by our family, by our cultural and religious environment, by our educational and political environment, by the western versus the eastern context, by the technological era, and so on. It is important to understand what has influenced, moulded and conditioned us. Through working with his cancer patients, Dr B. Siegel has noticed in his practice that 'negative conditioning is all too common...conditioning is at least as much a factor as genetic predisposition'.[9] And, to paraphrase Dr Siegel, I have observed in my practice that for people suffering from persistent fatigue, energy-draining conditioning is at least as much a risk factor in auto-immune disease as their genetic predispositions.

Health professionals must often face the beliefs related to the disabilities of a patient struggling with an illness, especially if this illness has long-term repercussions on his daily life. On a spiritual level, a list of patients' various perceptions of disabilities has been organized by Mary Ann McColl:[10] as an expression of divine will, as an opportunity for redemption, as a mission, as a punishment for sin, as a reminder of embodiment, as a condition of life, or as a combination of these perceptions. The temporary or permanent disability, as a consequence of the illness, forces us to face our finality, namely, death. We are consequently led to reflect on what is important to us. For many people, this observation results in a major overhaul of habits, relationships and work conditions. What can be achieved for some is an improved quality of daily life based on core values. For others, the end result will be one of denial and behaviours leading to an exacerbation of symptoms and a deep numbing of the senses.

Exercise 11.1: The link

The meaning that activities and occupations bring to your life is important. To find meaning in your present situation, observe the different types of conditioning that you have become internalized. First, for every theme suggested in Table 11.1, write down phrases that come to mind, phrases that you have often heard in your life, even more so if they have significantly influenced you from your childhood onwards, and those that have influenced you and that continue to feed the reflex loops in your thoughts. Anything is appropriate: a publicity slogan, a reproach from a parent, lyrics of a song, a proverb often used in your presence...

To put yourself more in context, take the time to read the different themes of conditioning in Table 11.2 in which several energizing and energy-draining phrases are listed, drawn from North American social conditioning – phrases often heard during a therapy session. This will give you an idea of the subtleties that can influence your behaviour.

TABLE 11.1 **Memes: beliefs, concepts, ideas, and other viruses of the mind**

THEMES	BELIEFS AND CONDITIONING
Body	
Illness	
Men versus women	
Expression of emotions	
Knowledge	
Relationship with others	
Relationship with oneself	
Time	
Money	
Work	
Leisure	
Change	
Spirituality	

TABLE 11.2 Current beliefs and conditioning

ENERGY-DRAINING	ENERGIZING
BODY	
The body is a sin. Overweight people are losers who lack self-discipline. Signs of ageing should be concealed to continue to be successful. We can no longer find a job at 50 years old. His back hurts; anything to avoid having to work. I will rest only when I'm finished. Medication is the only solution to my pain.	My body is a wonderful expression of creation. The body is the temple of the mind. Eating well is respecting yourself. I rest when I need to. I eat well to feel better. If I feel pain, I wonder about the cause. If I find the cause, I can possibly stop it to avoid suffering more.
EXPRESSION OF EMOTIONS	
Aggressiveness is acceptable for men. Men don't cry. She cries because she's a woman. Men can only express emotion amongst themselves in an athletic context. It is not acceptable to express our feelings in public.	Laughter is the way to true love. It is important to express yourself in order to change an uncomfortable situation. Directly explain what you are feeling without blaming others. In this way, they will be able to better understand you. If you have a problem with someone, it's with that person that you should resolve it.
KNOWLEDGE	
Nowadays, you need to study for a long time in order to succeed. I think therefore I am. She's only a mother…all she does is look after the kids! Without a degree, you can't find a job.	You can be what you want. Every human being has unique value. I am what I am and I'm proud of who I am. It's when ideas stop spinning inside my head that I find the best ideas. I am more efficient when I only do one thing at a time. Accumulation of knowledge is not knowledge.
OUR RELATIONSHIP WITH OTHERS	
We should always do our best. I only do what I'm told to do. But what are others going to think? We should sacrifice ourselves for a good cause. Honour thy father and thy mother. You must obey your parents. Respect no longer exists.	The more one pleases everybody, the less one pleases profoundly (Stendhal). Well-ordained charity starts with ourselves (from medieval Latin). I am responsible for all my choices. We harvest what we have sown. Help yourself and heaven will help you. Faithfulness starts with faithfulness to ourselves. Honour yourself.

WORK AND PLEASURE	
Work is not a pleasure!	Work is often the creator of pleasure.
We only work because we have to.	To work is to pray.
It's a sacrifice working day to day.	Working does not kill anybody.
We work only to pay taxes.	The harvest stems more from work than it
Job security prevails over the choice of	does from the fields.
work we love to do.	Keep an interest in your own career, how-
Work, work, work every day and every night.	ever humble.
Success is 10 per cent inspiration and 90	Failure does not exist. There are only
per cent perspiration.	mistakes that are opportunities to learn and
Only lazy people take naps.	grow.
Coffee breaks are a waste of time and of	When we set realistic guidelines we are
productivity.	respecting ourselves.
SPIRITUALITY	
God punishes.	Union is strength.
There is nothing after death.	In the universe, everything is interconnected.
Religion is obsolete! Believing in God is	God created us free.
for the imbeciles.	Life is a gift.
I put my life in the hands of God.	We are the expression of the energy in the
It is important for me to do everything by	Universe.
myself.	If God is Everything, we are a part of the
Nowadays, it's each one for himself.	Whole.
We are always alone in the world.	God is pure energy.
Life is a long struggle.	Life is a miracle.

Exercise 11.2: Power or powerlessness

Energy is power. Not having energy makes us unable to exert our power. It may mean that we do not want to be responsible or make a choice in a particular situation...

In the Energy Balance Sheet exercise in Chapter 3 you observed your way of behaving, during certain activities, based on the criteria of *powerlessness* or *power*. For each activity you checked off as powerlessness, try to find the belief underlying your behaviour. The list that you have already prepared can help you to establish relationships. Also identify the situations during which you feel energy or a certain form of *power*. Ask yourself if certain energy-draining beliefs could be modified to help you in this process and enable you to rediscover your power. Dare to modify your inner speech. Don't be afraid to put your beliefs to the test: transform these energy-draining beliefs into a source of healing energy. Write down this new perception under *Change of belief.* Use Table 11.3, as it will help you in your process.

For every activity next to which you ticked *powerlessness,* allow yourself to let go a little more, now that you are aware of the valuable energy you lose for no other reason than conditioning. Then dare to be a little more yourself. Let yourself *be.* Enter your new approach under the column 'I dare to...' Then evaluate the impact on your energy level once again, your change in perspective, going from powerlessness to power. Here are some suggestions that generate a feeling of power during an activity.

- Dare to be creative in what you do, say or the way you are.
- Dare to use your aesthetic sense.
- Dare to do an activity in a cheerful, playful way.
- Dare to feel kindness, without any self-deprecating thoughts in the back of your mind.
- Dare to be generous with yourself and others.
- Dare to accept praise and appreciation.
- Dare to allow room for others, let others help you in their own way rather than the way you would want the task to be done.
- Dare to say 'no'.
- Dare to allow others to be idle around you.
- Accept events as they come without judging them as good or bad.
- Accept your own current limitations, your fatigue and your aches and pains but without resignation.
- Dare to show gratitude every opportunity you are given to appreciate what life has to offer.
- Dare to be humble...not wanting to control everything all the time...dare to let go.

Once you have given yourself the right to change your perspective during your various activities, it will be easier for you to dare. As a result, you will be able to do the following:

- Dare to take some time for you alone.
- Dare to get closer to Nature to recharge your batteries, away from technology, so you can maintain the bond that connects you to the harmony of Nature.
- Dare to take ten minutes morning and evening to train your awareness and eventually your consciousness, using a technique of

your choice: meditation, observation of nature (walking in a park, gazing at a sunset, listening to the morning bird song), engage in one daily activity, mindfully, as suggested in Chapter 8: playing a musical instrument, eating a meal, folding clothes, dancing… Meditation can be done through activities. It only requires being mindful in the present moment by paying attention to what is really happening, here and now, and responding in a well thought-out manner rather than by just reacting to the illusions and the restlessness of the actual thinking. This is called contemplation.

The following are two examples taken from daily life.

Grocery shopping

- *Behaviour:* I buy my groceries as quickly as I can, in a very efficient way. I pick up my voicemail messages while I wait at the cash. I complain to myself that there are not enough cashiers.

- *Belief:* I have to be efficient at all costs. I have no spare time.

- *Change of belief:* It is important that I take care of myself. I am an important person in my life.

- *I dare to…* take my time doing the grocery shopping, noticing that I now have more energy to do it. I appreciate the time I spend waiting in line, which allows me to take a few mindful breaths and be aware of my bodily sensations. I also appreciate the fact that I do not have to use the self-serve cashier, as I am then able to smile at the cashier and have a light conversation with her as she smiles back at me.

Energy effect: ↑.

Talking to my boss about my work overload

- *Behaviour:* I take care of the work overload rather than ask for help. I avoid my boss because I am frustrated at having such a heavy workload. I am furious at my boss because he doesn't seem to understand that there's a problem — even though I haven't let him know that one exists (I have a passive attitude).

- *Belief:* Only the weak and the lazy complain to their boss. If I express myself, nobody will listen to me.

- *Change of belief:* I am a competent and efficient employee. I am neither lazy nor incapable. I am a valuable person and I respect my limitations. My colleagues aren't aware of any problems I'm having because I don't voice any. I have the right to express how I feel.

TABLE 11.3 I dare to…

ACTIVITIES	BEHAVIOUR: FORCED OR PASSIVE	BELIEF	MODIFICATION OF THE INITIAL BELIEF	I DARE TO…	ENERGY EFFECT (↑↓)

- *I dare to…* write out on a piece of paper what my problems are with the workload in order to clarify my thoughts instead of reacting to the situation; speak to my boss about the problems I am having; say 'no' to the excessive workload (I assert myself).

Energy effect: ↑.

Having some meaning in one's life, however tenuous, provides hope and courage to break through despair and loneliness often encountered in our clients. Lack of meaning of life, spiritual malaise or anomie, is manifested through loneliness, depression, sometimes anxiety and feelings of powerlessness.[12]

E. Townsend *et al.*

Summary

The occupational therapist knows that each daily activity is therapeutic in itself, that there is no dichotomy between work and personal life because the occupation (*ergon*) encompasses all activities: from working to brushing our teeth, having meals, taking the kids to school, giving hugs, tickles, having the giggles, etc. It's up to you to find energizing meaning in each of these activities. This will enable you to rediscover your power. Finding a personal and gratifying meaning in each thing, in every environment, and in every daily activity is a wonderful gift we all have.

A little inner voice, generated by your mind, may tell you that you don't have the time, that it's pointless, that it's only crap, or that it's unrealistic. If you believe that life is meaningless, why not create meaning? Why persist in 'forcing', in denying, in not using your imagination to give your life meaning, regardless of your reality, and regardless of the problems you have to deal with? Don't you deserve better than that? It's up to you to observe your resistance. Go back to the breathing rhythm and observe. Allow each breath to indicate what is occurring in the mind-body, and then experiment in several ways to rediscover your power. You will realize that time is created when we take the time to be, and that well-being settles in when we accept what is – without resigning ourselves. You will realize that after having observed these pains, fears, and emotions that, in the initial phase, often become more acute, such pains, fears, and emotions end up diminishing and even disappearing entirely. Continue to breathe and observe. It's possible that this observation will bring you to a state of well-being, and it will be sufficient. It's also possible, if you go deeper, that you will find your true *essence*, your *vitality* interconnected with the cosmos, and that you will feel the resulting *serenity*.

When your resistance dissipates, you will more easily agree to reserve a place for silence and daily meditation. Meditation, or a certain quality of presence, is a tool used to better know who we are; it demands nothing other than the desire to take the time to be, in all circumstances and during any activity. It is up to you to find your personal approach to life.

Mindful body sensation through movements (kinaesthesia)
in pleasant activities brings a sense of awareness
that helps restore our inner body harmony.

Chapter 12

Therapies and Therapists

Descartes said: 'I think, therefore I am.' Some traditions might say: 'I do not think, therefore the I or Self is.' Which point of 'you' is Truth?

The modern human's handicap

When I think of what most of us face during a day, of the nervous imbalance induced by the environment, and of our perception of this imbalance, which influences our body's entire musculature, I imagine the sketch in Figure 12.1.

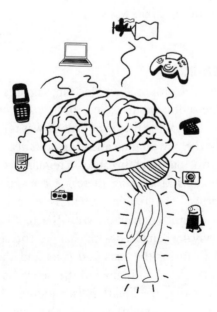

FIGURE 12.1 The modern human's handicap

I see an enormous neocortex endowed with a potential possessed by no other animal species. This brain is connected to multiple-interface extensions that intensify the incessant flow of info-energy that travels towards us at a dizzying speed, in real time. This brain must continuously adapt to new, increasingly sophisticated technologies, which force us to realize, more and more frequently, just how obsolete our acquired habits have become. The brain grows tired of creating effective loops of learning, but it does not have the time to delegate them long enough to the more automatic functions of the lower circuits. It therefore cannot create the habits that become anchored in our everyday life. As a result, the brain loses its relaxation mechanisms: sense of calm, restorative sleep, neurovegetative rhythms, and a feeling of inner well-being. It also loses the ability to observe before acting and to respond in a thoughtful manner, fully aware of the cause, as opposed to always 'acting' and 'reacting' in the same way. Memory needs time and rhythm because the faster the speed, the less we retain and the more exhausted we become. The autonomic nervous system (ANS) needs to slow down to be able to self-regulate. However, the brain is constantly hearing the same old story: 'You don't have time. You have to change, adapt, adjust your approach based on new interfaces.' But at what cost?

In order to gain a better understanding, let's take a brief look at how the various levels of our brain work.

The three brains

The *triune brain* model, proposed by Maclean, suggests that there are three brain levels.[1] The oldest brain, called the *reptilian brain*,[2] preceded the human brain and that of the first mammals. It was followed by the *limbic brain* and, finally, the new brain, called the *neocortex*. The reptilian brain is used for survival purposes because it regulates the neurovegetative system that maintains *homeostasis*: these are the functions of the ANS, as discussed earlier. The limbic system is in charge of adaptation. It therefore has a tight connection with the reptilian brain, which is motivated by survival when faced with change. This second evolutionary level, described as being the *emotional brain* and the *learning centre*, is located between the reptilian brain and the neocortex. The neocortex is considered the thinking headquarters (see Figure 12.2). Since survival takes precedence over thought (reason), the human brain must first ensure survival. Afterwards, if survival is achieved, the brain can think and reflect. In other words, after having run to seek refuge, we can think of a better way of acting next time: *respond rather than react.*

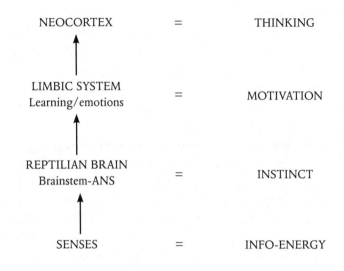

FIGURE 12.2 **The triune brain**

When the limbic system is drawn into the whirlwind of unlimited reflex adaptation, as previously described, messages from the body–mind, which describe emotions, are not heard clearly because we allow ourselves to be distracted by the excessive frequencies that blur the signals. This triggers derailment of the ANS, in which each movement, thought or sensory expression is perceived unconsciously, in a more heightened manner than usual, frequently resulting in reactions of *fight or flight.*

Independent of the cause of *persistent fatigue*, the body–mind disconnection can only intensify what the person is suffering from. In addition to being overburdened by the storage of blocked emotions, the body is thrown off balance by work and by the restricted and repetitive work habits. Potential outcomes include painful muscles that are no longer able to relax, particularly those activated by the cranial nerves, resulting in a constant tension in the jaw, shoulders, and throat, often causing postural, energy-draining deviations. An over-usage of certain muscle groups at the expense of other muscles generates micro-traumas, followed by tendinitis, bursitis, even displacement of the spine and the jaw joints. People who have already suffered from orthopaedic or congenital problems find themselves in an even more fragile state.

Energy efficiency

Perception and action are observed as being a continuum of a single process. If we tamper with perception, then action will be affected. In other words, if we modify our thinking, we will affect our actions, and if we modify the quality of our movements and our daily gestures, the quality of our perception will in turn be modified. We will see that one of these choices, when possible, is more energizing than the other.

As I have observed in my clients with neurological legions, the rehabilitation methods that use thinking (neocortex skills) are useful for bringing certain favourable changes to an energy-draining dysfunction: these methods are referred to as compensatory. However, they themselves are energy-draining and gradually become less efficient as the individual grows increasingly tired during the day. When a person uses these techniques, he must think in each stage of the activity he does because his automatic circuit loops are deficient.

Top-down compensatory methods refer to the use of conscious thinking during the sequence of an activity, which normally occurs automatically as a result of circuits reinforced by experience at a sub-cortical level. These are subtle adjustments that would normally be made unconsciously and which are, according to this practice, implemented by the brain's conscious functions. This process is highly energy-draining. We fruitlessly give the same instructions to the patient so he learns how to compensate, only to have old, less effective approaches reappear at the end of the day or when a common cold emerges from a stressful situation (the child who has a learning disability starts to make the same writing mistakes again; the foot of the hemiplegic leg starts to drag along the ground while walking; the teenager who has been told many times to sit up straight reverts to slouching, etc.).

To visualize the principle, let's imagine a context in which the captain of a large fifteenth-century three-mast ship is the neocortex and that he gives orders to his junior, subcortical crew members who are at their posts, each performing a very specific task. Each crew member carries out his work automatically. The tasks have become so simple due to years and years of repeating the same tasks: tying knots, hoisting the sails, maintaining the deck in response to different weather conditions, etc.

In this context, the top-down method advocates that, instead of enlisting inexperienced seamen and teaching them how to do certain tasks, the captain will carry out all the work, even if he is already busy dealing with his own responsibilities at the helm of the marine sextant. If only one experienced man was lacking, the captain could possibly step in, but this wouldn't be an effective way of delegating work. However, if an insufficient or unqualified crew was facing a dangerous situation, of course the captain should assist his men to return to port. Hence the purpose of the top-down method.

There is another, more energizing, choice that incorporates both the nautical example and that of the brain of exhausted people: the *bottom-up* learning method. In contrast to the top-down method, this method aims to stimulate the subcortical functions so they themselves can carry out the repetitive work and make the unconscious adjustments. As a result, the neocortex gives the orders and takes care of other tasks in which it excels, rather than executing the order itself. On our large ship, it would be better to recruit a deck boy so he could do what he was taught without having to ask for assistance from the captain. And it would be logical for the captain to find new crew members to replace those who are injured or absent – rather than taking on the work for them.

In this chapter I will briefly list certain types of therapy and provide an overview of a choice of exercises and activities intended to optimize the possibility of rehabilitation, while promoting energy efficiency. In the choice of interventions, I will address the different ways of paying interest on the energy debt, while conserving the most acquired capital possible to promote the body's natural self-healing.

It is important to find activities that favour the body's reappropriation through the senses and bodily movements: this is what I previously described when I was speaking about therapies based primarily on the bottom-up theory. The suggested techniques have therefore been selected according to the following hypothesis: regaining balance through unconscious, automatic, and preconscious subcortical functions of the reptilian brain, of the cerebellum and of the basal nuclei (bottom-up method). This approach, more economical from an energy perspective, is preferable to the acquisition of compensatory techniques that immediately enlist the neocortex (top-down method).

Activities

Your daily life is your temple and your religion.
When you enter into it take with you your all.

Khalil Gibran

I am currently using my occupational therapist's perception to propose suggestions to you in an effort to promote well-being and, if possible, to assist you in the natural healing process that we all deal with. This hardly replaces the consultation with an occupational therapist who knows you and who could help you to adapt your activities based on your needs, but it is a starting point on the journey that could be done without assistance. I have selected activities that reestablish the balance in your PNI system. I will also explain how to become aware of how you behave in your daily activities so as to make them not only more efficient and harmonious, but more meaningful and, as a result, energizing. Don't forget that it's as much the *context* (*your point of view*) as the *content* (*the activity*) that will foster your well-being and, perhaps, your healing process.

My professional interest in treatment techniques applied to neurological diseases has led me to choose activities that follow the human being's sensory-motor development. I couldn't help but observe in my quest for potential solutions that the PNI balance is influenced by bodily movements and that a less energy-draining posture is re-established. Harmony and efficiency of these bodily movements develop following the child's stages of development.

When ANS is compared to a vehicle's brake and accelerator pedals, it can be said that we are once again teaching the body to use the brake pedal to reestablish the rhythms of the parasympathetic functions, and that we are also reteaching the body to slow down by gradually lifting the foot off the accelerator, too often fully floored against the sympathetic functions.[3] In both cases, we put ourselves in efficiency mode from an energy perspective, but in different ways: the first restores and regenerates the PNI super-system, while the second stops spending unnecessarily.

Another criterion has led me to choose activities that stimulate the retraining of specific reflex loops in a playful, calm, parasympathetic environment and, of course, in a context in which the pace of the movements fosters this approach and leaves the neocortex in peace to continue at its own duties as master mariner. Thanks to these techniques, the neocortex has ample time to explore new continents of knowledge, rather than compensating for the gaps caused by the loops of energy-draining automatic movements/thoughts.

Restoring the body–mind balance through activity

The cultivation of the energy in the fluidity of taiji movements
is meant to be carried through daily activities as well.

I am proposing a list of methods that will enable you to rebalance your ANS based on your energy level. The benefits of these methods have been scientifically tested. I have often used them in my practice. Other methods, which are also beneficial, have been added. From the list, choose the one (or ones) that suit you and take the necessary steps to adequately use it (them).

To rebalance the body–mind, it is important to gradually increase the energy demand based on your energy level, which you can assess by referring to the Daily Energy Scale (DES) in Appendix 5, and in Table 4.1. If you are uncertain of your energy level, start with a light activity (from 2 to 3 METS) and *gradually* increase the intensity. If you decide to go for a walk, go slowly, for 10 minutes, and then increase to 15, then to 20 minutes. If your body can tolerate exercise, increase the speed at which you walk. The energy demand will then reach a moderate level (4 to 5 METS). I don't suggest any maximum-intensity activity during the rehabilitation phase, at least not until you have reached 70 per cent on your DES, over at least three consecutive days. Your level of fatigue or abnormal pain, or both, immediately after exercise or the next day, will be your guide as to whether to increase (or not) the intensity of physical exercise.

The lying down position

- *Hypnosis:*[4] Call upon a psychologist certified to perform hypnosis or another health professional with an expertise in visualization. They can perform personalized recordings in order to favourably influence the balance of your ANS.[5]

- *Autosuggestion and visualization:* If you have limited financial means and you have adequate concentration to perform your own autosuggestion exercises, I suggest that you read the book by Shakti Gawain, *Creative Visualization*.[6] This book proposes a variety of brief energizing visualization exercises that regulate breathing and ANS.

- *Relaxation method:* The method I mainly use with my clients who are anxious, depressed or who suffer from neurological diseases, is the Schulz method of autogenous relaxation.[7] Insist that your therapist focus on the musculature of the face and neck, which are primarily activated by the cranial nerves. This method consists in mentally relaxing each part of the body. Those with smaller budgets should realize that this type of effective tool is available on CD, however the CD cannot replace an experienced therapist.

- *Acupuncture:* Acupuncture has been a part of traditional Chinese medicine (TCM) treatments for several millenia. It is well known for treating pain, but it does a lot more than that: it acts in various ways on the PNI system. Many of its health benefits have been scientifically proved.[8]

- *Heart coherence:* Several authors suggest this method that also has the effect of rebalancing the ANS.[9] It has a significant favourable effect on anxiety, depression, and cardiac problems. You can now find professionals trained in this field. Information on this method can be found through the Institute of Heart Math (www. heartmath.org).

- *Massage therapy:* We can choose from different types of massage. A relaxation massage can help you in your approach to life, because it promotes abdominal breathing and saves energy. Massage reduces the rate of stress hormones and increases the neuropeptides of the reward circuit and of well-being.[10] A massage can be a wise choice, but enquire about its therapeutic effects. Touching between lovers and signs of affection between parents and children bring many benefits to the recipient and to the giver,[11] and they have the *added bonus* of being free.

- *The EMDR technique,* described by Dr Servan-Schreiber,[12] is an effective method if you want to adjust an inadequate reflex loop caused by a particularly traumatic past event.

Gradual transition from a reclining to standing position

- *Meditation:* The word 'meditation' – like the words 'medicine' and 'medication' – comes from the Latin *meditari*, iterative of *mederi*, which means 'to care'. The latest research shows that supporters of meditation keep themselves in a highly regenerative state for the sake of their brain. Davidson's research confirms the previous research that emphasizes activity performed by the left prefrontal cortex during meditation, the region that is associated with energizing emotions and thoughts.[13] The mindfulness meditation stress-management groups have proven that they are highly beneficial for those in favour of this type of approach.[14]

- *The Feldenkrais method* is a form of somatic education (related to the senses) developed by the engineer of that name following a knee injury, and triggered by his curiosity about the science of the human body.[15] To find a qualified professional, contact the association or guild in your area.[16] The purpose of this technique is to become reconnected to our body–mind, and this is possible through gentle movements carried out and guided by the therapist. This technique improves the quality of movement, decreases tension, lengthens the musculature, reduces pain and heightens body awareness (kinaesthesis).[17] It can be practised in a group setting.

- *Traditional stretching:*[18] Stretches are beneficial for releasing tension and relaxing the muscles and they help to eliminate the toxins trapped in the muscles (lactic acid) and in the lymphatic system. Choose a method that you are already familiar with rather than reinventing the wheel. Yoga stretches are very effective if they are done gently, without forcing the body to hold an uncomfortable position.[19] If you have experienced stiffness, pain, and tension for a long time, or if you suffer from arthritis, a few physiotherapy sessions could help you effectively avoid injuries triggered by inadequate or inappropriate stretches.

- *Padovan Method®:* This method of neurofunctional reorganization was developed by Beatrice Padovan, speech pathologist. It is based on movements linked to the neurological organization in relation to the sensory motor development milestone of childhood. I favour this method in my practice because it stimulates many functions activated by cranial nerves, which share a direct link with the reptilian brain. Moreover, it stimulates proper reflex activity (following the bottom-up principle), provides direct stimulation to some parasympathetic rhythms described in Chapter 7, and includes rhythmic movements recapitulating motor development movements. If you are interested in knowing more about this method, contact the resource in your area.[20] After using this method, immediately after the first session, I noticed a change in all my patients suffering from persistent fatigue with various diagnoses – and even in people who had been on work stoppage for several years.

- *Singing:* It is free and stimulates the parasympathetic branch of the ANS in many ways. It regulates abdominal breathing while stimulating the tongue and pharynx muscles (activated by several cranial nerves with a parasympathetic component); it activates other cranial nerves by stimulating the facial and throat muscles; and it stimulates the secretion of saliva, while promoting nasal breathing and soft palate movement, like yawning (a parasympathetic response). All this prepares the ear for the rhythm of the music, which influences the heart rate. Choose energizing songs with a repetitive hopeful theme and sing along with your favourite artists. When we sing we live in the here and now and fill our lungs with oxygen while having fun! It puts a smile on the faces of children, colleagues, and even people who catch a glimpse of you singing while you drive!

- *Qi Gong and taiji:*[21] These millennial techniques, both based on TCM principles,[22] demonstrate the effective wisdom of returning to a calm state, to an approach of conscious and controlled breathing, and to a body awareness and a fine-tuning of the senses, particularly the kinaesthetic sense (our position in space while we move).[23] The most exhausted people (40% and less on the DES) will benefit more from Qi Gong (taiji is more demanding). A qualified teacher can nevertheless adapt taiji techniques to a seated position. I would always begin my *persistent fatigue pain and stress management* workshops with a Qi Gong exercise.[24] My patients really appreciate these exercises, because their powerful effect brings them into the present moment. With respect to taiji, I recommend Chan Ssu Chin exercises, in which the movement is an end in itself, rather than a choreography, which ends up being too energy-draining for those who have been exhausted for a long time. Fortunately, these exercises can easily be modified based on individual needs.

- *Recreation that brings you pleasure:* Reading a novel, a magazine, playing a musical instrument, attending a concert or a show, painting, doing crochet, wood work, and gardening, are activities that bring pleasure and relieve tension. The playful attitude plays a key role in the meaning that is attributed to activities. It promotes a tolerant attitude with regard to change, increases the ability to face difficult situations and improves health and well-being.[25] The playful attitude stems from a perception of the activity that stimulates *reward circuits* rather than *punishment circuits*, which we discussed in Chapter 9.

Standing position

- *Walking:* Going for a walk with sharp senses (like in the exercises of Chapter 8) and with an awareness of movements, breathing and the support of the heel on the ground before the sole of the foot will help you to stay grounded in the present. And there are other things to discover! Trees, squirrels, birds, the changing seasons... and even mushrooms!

- *Visualization exercise while walking:* If the incessant flow of thoughts overwhelms you and you don't know how to be when you go for a walk, I suggest that you choose one of the following dualities and pronounce these words at the rhythm of your breathing. This will free you from the reflex loops of thoughts that assault you. Don't pronounce all the affirmations on the same walk, a single one is enough. If it helps you, add a second one, but no more. One affirmation per month is enough to encourage the appearance of new, pleasant reflex loops.

Each time you exhale...	*Each time you inhale...*
...I expel discomfort.	*...I feel healthy.*
...anger vanishes.	*...serenity takes over.*
...pain dissipates.	*...well-being takes its place.*
...sadness leaves.	*...I'm filled with joy.*
...dispair disappears.	*...hope appears.*
...doubt fades.	*...confidence grows.*
...unconsciousness is unlocked.	*...consciousness is raised.*

- *Dance:* If you enjoy musical rhythms and music relaxes you, know that dancing is a very good way to make your body vibrate harmoniously. Start with soft music and observe your tolerance to this activity. It's up to you to determine the rhythm that suits you and the duration of the dance. Let yourself go.

- *Swimming:* Movements carried out in the water are excellent, even if you only walk, float, or move. I recommend swimming in natural water, in lakes, rivers, and the sea. If you suffer from environmental sensitivities (described in Chapter 2), you may react to the chlorine used in public pools. If this is the case, avoid swimming. The rhythmic movements of the crawl, backstroke, and breaststroke synchronize with the breathing and have a regulating effect on the ANS.

- *Cycling:* Here again, rhythm associating breathing with movement has a regulating effect on the ANS. However, the energy demand for such an activity could be too high with respect to your current recovery level. Check this by referring to the DES. Start by pedalling along a flat surface, rather than by wanting to conquer an incline. The zen advice of 'no goal, no profit' is important for regulating the PNI system: choose to go on a bicycle ride rather than throwing yourself into a race against the clock. The point, with cycling as with the previous activities, is to maintain a constant pace in order to promote the body's internal regulation.

Summary

I do not recommend any intense physical activity in this book, and I suggest, before getting back into shape, you have your abilities assessed by an occupational therapist or a physiotherapist. They will indicate the best approach to take. Don't forget that, when there is inactivity, the muscles 'deflate' in less than two weeks, and the body needs gradual training to get back into shape. The areas of muscular and postural imbalance must be corrected before you embark on more rigorous activities; don't move furniture or do a big spring clean without training beforehand! If you have developed an auto-immune disease, make sure you are monitored by a doctor who listens and with whom you can discuss your abilities.

At the risk of repeating myself, it is important to move rhythmically to encourage self-regulation of the body–mind and self-healing. It is also imperative to stretch to activate the circulation and prevent acid and free radicals from accumulating and stagnating. It is therefore highly important to choose one or two methods that get you moving, despite fatigue and pain and that respect your limits. Seek the help of a healthcare professional if you feel you are not able to make the choices by yourself. Graduate the duration of your activity before increasing its intensity. Integrate the activity into your lifestyle so it becomes a habit, either on a daily basis or several times a week. It's up to you to make choices based on your personality, your state of health, and your financial resources.

Chapter 13

Adrenal Glands

In Traditional Chinese Medicine, the adrenal glands are part of the kidney organ system, which is known as the Root of Life.

Although the entire endocrine system is overworking throughout the PNI imbalance, the adrenal glands play a key role in responding to stressors. For information purposes, I am going to touch briefly on the functions of these stressors so we can understand some of the symptoms of PNI imbalance listed in Chapter 1.

The adrenal glands resemble two small pyramids perched on the kidneys.[1] They are composed of two sections: the outer part, which is called the cortex, and the centre, which is called the medulla. In fact, these two sections are two separate endocrine glands: the medulla, which works like a modified sympathetic ganglion and the cortex, which is divided into four sections. The medulla produces info-energy messengers called *catecholamines* (Table 13.1) and the cortex secretes *steroid* messengers[2] (Table 13.2).

TABLE 13.1 **Medulla and catecholamines**

HORMONES	ACTION
Epinephrine (80%)	Cardiovascular
	Central nervous system
	General metabolism
Norepinephrine	Cardiovascular
Enkephalins	Natural analgesics
Chromogranin A	Natural tranquilizer

TABLE 13.2 Adrenal cortex and steroid hormones

AREA	HORMONES
Zona reticularis and Interface zone	Pregnenolone Progesterone Oestrogens Testosterone Androsterones Andostenedione
Zona fasciculata (glucocorticoïdes)	Cortisol (hydrocortisone)
Zona glomerulosa (mineralocorticoids)	Aldosterone

Catecholamines are neurotransmitters and hormones that respond to *fight-or-flight* situations. In the nervous system, they 'electrically' act as neurotransmitters following the sympathetic pathways of the ANS and are alerted through neuronal connections linked to their 'controller,' the hypothalamus. They are also stimulated by the hormonal communication pathway from the hypothalamus to the adrenal glands (refer to Chapter 6, Figure 6.1). This communication pathway uses the blood vessels to reach the glands and is slower than the 'electrical' nervous pathway. These hormones originate from the same substance as the thyroid hormone, namely tyrosine (Figure 13.1).

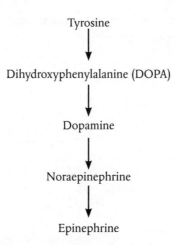

Tyrosine

↓

Dihydroxyphenylalanine (DOPA)

↓

Dopamine

↓

Noraepinephrine

↓

Epinephrine

FIGURE 13.1 Biosynthesis of catecholamines

Cholesterol is the substrate for the biosynthesis of all steroid hormones (refer to Figure 13.2): every hormone is interrelated to other hormones of which it is possibly the precursor. For example, to produce *cortisol*, *aldosterone*, and *oestrogens*, we need *cholesterol* transformed into *pregnenolone*, which will itself be transformed into progesterone. In stressful situations, we urgently require cortisol so we can make the hypothesis that this will have an impact on the production and the secretion of other hormones, such as oestrogens, testosterone, and aldosterone.

Other points to consider:

- Some hormones compete for the same cell receptors (like *cortisol* and *progesterone*), which disturbs the normal functioning of the latter if the first hormone (cortisol) is secreted in large amounts, which is what tends to occur when we find ourselves in a very stressful situation over a long period of time.

- It is now recognized that the xenohormones from the environment (refer to Chapter 2) have an oestrogenic effect on both genders.[3] According to Dr John Lee they create multiple endocrine disruptions by accumulating in target tissues over time.[4]

- If a specific catalyst is missing in the synthesis of one hormone to meet a very high demand, this can result in a greater PNI imbalance (e.g. vitamin B6, magnesium insufficiency).

- The inflammatory response increases cortisol and *oestrogen* levels but suppresses progesterone.[5]

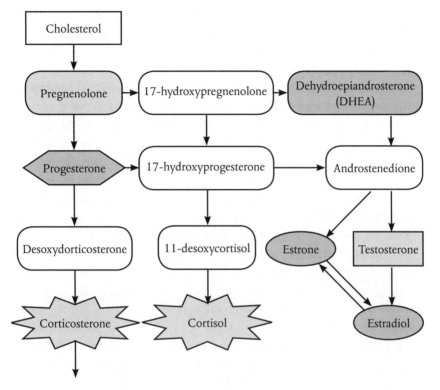

FIGURE 13.2 Biosynthesis of steroids[6]

The link between cortisol and insulin

Hormones shape behavioural response. Hungry people can be irritable due to their lower blood glucose level, which reflects hormonal adjustments. Early morning impatience can reflect the lower level of catecholamines and other hormones in the brain.

The way in which the blood sugar level regulates itself by the adrenal cortex is by secreting cortisol that raises its level in order to meet the energy demand, since glucose is the main substance used in creating cellular energy: this is referred to as a hyperglycaemic effect. Epinephrine and thyroxin (a thyroid hormone) also have a hyperglycaemic effect on blood glucose.[7] In the pancreas, glucagon also has a hyperglycaemic effect because it releases the glucose stored as glycogen in the liver into the blood stream:[8] this is called *glycogenolysis*.

Insulin is secreted in response to a high blood glucose concentration that can be triggered whenever stress or a high energy demand arises. It is the only hypoglycaemic hormone: it enables glucose to easily enter the cells. In the liver, insulin helps to store glucose as glycogen. It inhibits the production of glucose by reducing glycogenolysis. Inside the cells, it stimulates the uptake of glucose to produce energy through *glycolysis*. An increase in insulin secretion therefore causes hypoglycaemia and this decreased glucose level in the blood can be experienced in the body as a glandular stress that promotes further PNI imbalance.[9]

Tracking glucose: Glucose is easily absorbed through the small intestine and then travels through the portal venous system to the liver or another destination. Glucose can be transformed as a reserve (glycogenesis) in the liver. An increased blood sugar level caused by quick glucose absorption triggers a massive insulin secretion by the pancreas, which also excites the adrenal glands and consequently triggers secretion of hyperglycaemic hormones (cortisol and epinephrine). As a result, stress is felt throughout the entire PNI system, causing the *pancreas* and the *liver* to significantly step up their efforts. For many years, despite the repetitive attacks of refined and artificially engineered food, our body continues to maintain a balanced blood glucose level. Over time, the pancreas becomes exhausted and can no longer produce the required amount of insulin. A tired and abused pancreas leads to an auto-immune disease, namely, Type 2 diabetes.

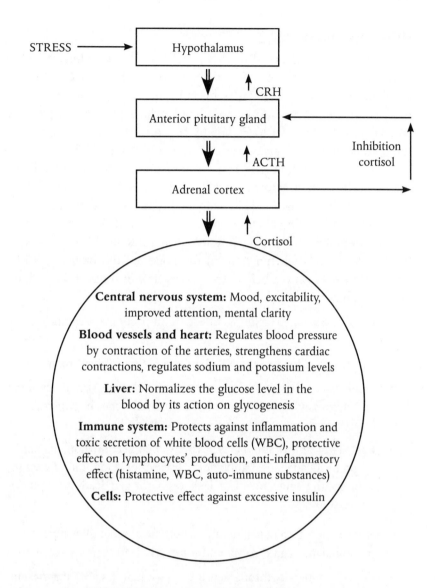

FIGURE 13.3 Hypothalamus-pituitary-adrenal axis

CRH = corticotrophin-releasing hormone
ACTH = corticotrophin

Hormonal imbalance

While the catecholamines of the ANS and the adrenal medulla stimulate target organs' reaction to fight or flee (Table 6.1), the brain, through the hypothalamus, sends its messengers to increase the adrenal cortisol production. We call this information complex the hypothalamus-pituitary adrenal axis (HPA) (refer to Figure 13.3). Cortisol becomes busy while responding to stress in many ways, as shown in Figure 13.3.

Aldosterone is a hormone that retains sodium (Na+) and releases potassium (K+) in an effort to regulate sodium and potassium levels in the body; it plays a major role in maintaining the body fluid balance and therefore in influencing blood pressure and cellular hydration. The other steroid hormones play many physiological roles in different systems but the details of their functions in the body are too numerous to be discussed here. However, here is a brief overview of some of their effects on the brain:

- *Progesterone* has a calming effect. It impacts every tissue of the body.

- *Dehydroepiandrosterone (DHEA)* gives a feeling of well-being.

- *Testosterone*, when produced in too high a dosage, stimulates anger and aggressivity. It is also associated with acne, hypoglycaemia, infertility, ovarian cysts, and increased body hair;

- Excess of *oestrogen* stimulates passivity, mental confusion, insomnia, migraine headaches, gallbladder disease, oedema, mood swings, and, by the same token, a lack of oestrogen leads to signs of depression.[10]

It is therefore logical to conclude that when the adrenal glands get tired, hormonal imbalance can directly and indirectly lead to:

- loss of minerals through urine – sodium (Na+), magnesium (Mg+), and potassium (K+) – that is felt as a craving for salt and eventually hypotension and dehydration

- an unstable blood glucose level (rollercoaster ride between hypo- and hyperglycemia), and eventually a lack of intracellular glucose, leading to persistent fatigue, and a lack of cerebral glucose, observed as a decrease in cognitive skills

- irregular menstrual cycle for women, erectile dysfunction for men and a change in libido for both sexes and a possible acne flair-up

- amplified inflammatory and immune responses (due to a lack of cortisol to modulate them)

- mood swings, depending on which hormone or hormone(s) are excessive or insufficient

- a deficiency of good *cholesterol* as a result of an inadequate diet (refer to Chapter 5) can lead to an aggravated hormonal imbalance

- since cortisol is toxic for the limbic brain when continuously produced in high amounts,[11] loss of working memory and other cognitive and mood disorders can be observed.

To give you a general idea of the complex interrelationships within the glandular system, here is a small example of what is observed more and more often in women suffering from persistent fatigue. When such women are menopausal or have luteal insufficiency (that is, they are approaching menopause and produce less *progesterone* through the reproductive system), the adrenal glands become the only source of progesterone. Adrenal insufficiency in this stage of a woman's life can heighten the symptoms of a PNI imbalance. Some women can even suffer from symptoms of hypothyroidism (see Appendix 1) at menopause.[12] Since the limbic system is part of the brain that receives the most thyroid hormones,[13] the decrease in the rate of this hormone has a negative effect on the production of several messengers of information, including serotonin, which contributes to depression when its production is low.

For those who want to learn more about the PNI system, I suggest several websites,[14] and several authors whose works are included in the References.[15] We have finally arrived at a crossroads of science at which the brain, the endocrine system and the immune system are considered as being the tripod of health. Einstein was possibly right when he said that 'The orthodox tendency to divide makes no sense…'

All the best on your journey!

Appendices

When you need to carry one of the Appendices around with you to refer to, you can download and print a copy from www.jkp.com/catalogue/book/9781848191013/resources.

Appendix 1: Comparative Symptoms

	HYPOGLYCAEMIA	ADRENAL FATIGUE	HYPOTHYROIDISM	HYPERTHYROIDISM	OESTROGEN DOMINANCE	DEPRESSION
COGNITIVE AND EMOTIONAL MANIFESTATIONS						
COGNITIVE	Trouble concentrating Forgetfulness Irritability Mental confusion	Trouble concentrating Forgetfulness Lack of mental clarity Irritability Mental confusion when rushed Decreased productivity (see Table 1.3)	Decreased attention Forgetfulness Irritability Audiovisual hallucinations	Irritability/aggression Feelings of guilt Mental disorganization	Memory gaps	Trouble concentrating Forgetfulness Indecisiveness Lack of self-esteem
EMOTIONAL	Depression	Inability to tolerate stress Feelings of despair Anxiety/fears	Depressive mood Lack of interest Loss of ambition Agoraphobia Emotional instability Paranoid ideation (in severe cases) Manic behaviour Dementia (in severe cases)	Depression Anxiety Night distress Panic attacks Lack of emotional control Paranoia	Depression Anxiety Emotional instability	Depressive mood, sadness Lack of interest or lack of pleasure Feelings of guilt Feelings of despair Suicidal thoughts or thoughts of death

	HYPOGLYCAEMIA	ADRENAL FATIGUE	HYPOTHYROIDISM	HYPERTHYROIDISM	OESTROGEN DOMINANCE	DEPRESSION
PHYSICAL MANIFESTATIONS						
GENERAL	Frequent headaches following alcohol consumption Sensitivity to noise Yawning or drowsiness	Frequent, often unexplained headaches Sleep disturbances			Headaches Acceleration of the ageing process Hypoglycaemia Insomnia	Insomnia or hypersomnia
EYES	Blurred vision Sensitivity to light			Eye irritation	Eye irritation Dry eyes	
SKIN	Cold hands and feet	A white line appears when skin is scratched Brown spots on the face, neck and shoulders Sensitivity to cold	Thickening of the skin Dry and pale skin Brittle hair Hair loss	Hives Brittle nails Itchiness Hair loss Intolerance to heat	Hair loss	
CIRCULATORY	Hypotension Dizziness Loss of consciousness Palpitations Shortness of breath Excessive sweating (at night)	Hypotension Dizziness Loss of consciousness Arrhythmia/palpitations Shortness of breath	Sensitivity to cold even when it is warm	Arrhythmia/palpitations Shortness of breath Chest pain Warm and sweaty hands	Increased blood clotting	
IMMUNE	Increased allergies More prone to respiratory tract infections	Swollen lymph nodes or swollen glands (neck area) Associated with auto-immune diseases More prone to respiratory tract infections			Associated with respiratory allergies and auto-immune diseases	

PHYSICAL MANIFESTATIONS						
GASTRO-INTESTINAL	Feeling of constant hunger Food cravings: chocolate, sugar, starch, etc. Weight loss or gain Nausea and vomiting with no apparent reason	Salt cravings Weight loss Digestive problems	Weight gain	Anaemia Large appetite Very thirsty Weight loss Frequent stools	Weight gain Bloating	Decreased or increased appetite Weight loss: more than 5% of weight
REPRODUCTIVE	Hot flashes	Exacerbated PMS (10 days) Decreased sexual desire	Heavy menstrual bleeding or amenorrhea	Breast enlargement in men (1/3)	PMS Irregular periods Infertility Decreased sexual desire Sensitive breasts (women) Ovarian cysts Cancer: uterus, breast, prostate Uterine fibroma Cervical dysplasia Early start of menstruation	Decreased sexual desire

	HYPOGLYCAEMIA	ADRENAL FATIGUE	HYPOTHYROIDISM	HYPERTHYROIDISM	OESTROGEN DOMINANCE	DEPRESSION
MUSCULO-SKELETAL	Lack of coordination Hand tremors when hungry Jerky movements Painful joints Weakness without any apparent reason Sudden energy drops Waking up tired Physical exhaustion	Tremors when tense Swollen ankles at night Agitated limbs Muscle weakness Sudden energy drops Persistent fatigue	Swollen extremities Hoarse voice Muscle cramps Painful joints and muscles General fatigue	Tremors Tongue tremors Psychomotor agitation Muscle weakness Fatigue Hyperactivity	Water retention Loss of bone mass Fatigue	Psychomotor agitation or retardation Fatigue or energy loss
ASSOCIATED DISEASES						
	Allergies Diabetes Selye's phase of exhaustion	Allergies Hypoglycaemia Multiple chemical sensitivities Respiratory diseases Rheumatoid arthritis Fibromyalgia Myalgic encephalomyelitis Other auto-immune diseases	Other auto-immune diseases	Anaemia Other auto-immune diseases	Gallbladder diseases Mimics hypothyroidism Magnesium deficiency Osteoporosis Breast cancer Prostate cancer Uterine cancer	

References

W. H. Philpott and D. K. Kalita, *Brain Allergies* (second edition), Chicago, Keats Publishing, 2000, p.148; Association des hypoglycémique du Québec, www.hypoglycemie.qc.ca/index.php?option=com_content&task=view&id=17&Itemid=32; James L. Wilson, *Adrenal Fatigue: The 21st Century Stress Syndrome*, Petaluma, CA, Smart Publications, 2001; J. Wass, S. Shalet, *Oxford Textbook of Endocrinology And Diabetes*. Bath, Oxford University Press, 2002; Arem Ridha, *The Thyroid Solution*, Toronto, Random House Publishing, 1999; J. Lee, J. Hanley, and V. Hopkins, *What Your Doctor Won't Tell You About Premenopause* New York, Warners Books, 1999; American Psychiatric Association, *Diagnostic and Statistical Manual of Mental Disorders* (4th edition), Washington, APA, 2000, pp.27–33.

Appendix 2A: Mineral Nutritional Deficiencies

	ADRENAL FATIGUE	MAGNESIUM (MG)	IRON (FE)	POTASSIUM (K)	CALCIUM (CA)	SELENIUM (SE)	ZINC (ZN)
COGNITIVE AND EMOTIONAL SYMPTOMS							
COGNITIVE	Trouble concentrating Forgetfulness Inability to think clearly Irritability Decreased productivity Mental confusion when rushed	Irritability Decreased productivity Nervousness	Memory loss Irritability Decreased productivity Mental confusion		Convulsions Mental confusion		
EMOTIONAL	Inability to tolerate stress Feelings of despair Anxiety/fears	Decreased resistance when fatigued Depression					
PHYSICAL SYMPTOMS							
GENERAL AND METABOLIC	Frequent, often unexplained headaches Sudden drop in energy Chronic fatigue Trouble sleeping	Early ageing process Chronic fatigue Reduced cellular metabolism Reduced ATP transformation	Chronic headaches Lack of energy Chronic fatigue	Fatigue		Obesity related to hypothyroidism	Growth delay
SKIN, NAILS, HAIR	A white line appears when the skin is scratched Brown spots appear on face, neck and shoulders	Tooth decay, more prone to dental cavities Brittle nails	Pale skin, especially in the facial area Tingling sensation in fingers or toes				Wounds heal slowly

	ADRENAL FATIGUE	MAGNESIUM (MG)	IRON (FE)	POTASSIUM (K)	CALCIUM (CA)	SELENIUM (SE)	ZINC (ZN)
VASCULAR	Sensitivity to cold Hypotension Dizziness Lack of consciousness Arrhythmic/palpitations	Myocarditis Linked with atherosclerosis Coronary lesions Tachycardia	Sensitivity to cold Dizziness Shortness of breath	Cardiac diseases Arrhythmia	Hypertension Arrhythmia	Cardiac diseases Kashin's disease	
IMMUNE	Swollen lymph nodes (in the neck or in the neck glands) Associated with auto-immune diseases Catches colds easily	Reduced phagocytosis Inflammation Oxydation Weakened resistance to disease and infections Catches colds easily	Increased risk of infections				Reduced immune functions
GASTRO-INTESTINAL	Trouble digesting Salt cravings Weight loss	Loss of appetite Nausea Vomiting Decreased bile secretions Decreased pancreatic and intestinal secretions	Loss of appetite Weight loss Trouble swallowing Cancer sores Painful and/or swollen tongue Need to drink cold water, bite ice cubes	Intestinal sluggishness Bloating Abdominal pain Constipation	Loss of appetite		
REPRODUCTIVE AND URINARY	Exacerbated PMS (10 days) Decreased sexual desire	PMS Painful uterine contractions A cause of renal stones Contributes to prostatic oedema	Heavy menstrual bleeding prior to iron deficiency symptoms				

MUSCULO-SKELETAL	Tremors: *When tense* Swollen ankles at night Agitated limbs Muscle weakness	Tremors: *Spasmophilia, tetany* Oedema Muscle cramps Numbness Tingling Muscle weakness	Muscle weakness	Muscle cramps Muscle weakness	Prone to fractures Numbness Tingling Muscle cramps Decrease in bone mass		Restless leg syndrome
OTHER ASSOCIATED CONDITIONS	Allergies Multiple chemical sensitivities Respiratory diseases Rheumatoid arthritis Fibromyalgia Other immune and auto-immune diseases	Allergies and intolerances due to decreased phagocytosis Associated with modern diseases Decreased resistance to stress			Decreased bone density (osteopenia) Osteoporosis	Hypothyroidism Kashin-Beck disease (osteoarthropathy)	

Appendix 2B: Nutritional Deficiencies – Hydrosoluble Vitamins

	ADRENAL FATIGUE	THIAMINE B1 DEFICIENCY	RIBOFLAVIN B2 DEFICIENCY	NIACIN NICOTINA-MIDE B3 DEFICIENCY	PENTATONIC ACID B5 DEFICIENCY	PYRIDOXINE B6 DEFICIENCY	FOLIC ACID B9 DEFICIENCY	CYANOCO-BALAMIN B12 DEFICIENCY	VITAMIN C DEFICIENCY
COGNITIVE AND AFFECTIVE MANIFESTATIONS									
COGNITIVE	Decreased concentration Forgetfulness Does not think clearly Irritability Decreased productivity Mental confusion when stressed	Polyneuritis Mental confusion			Neurological problems Paraesthesia Tingling	Neurological problems Irritability	Forgetfulness Irritability Mood swings	Demyelination Forgetfulness Confusion Balance problems	
EMOTIONAL	Feelings of despair Inability to tolerate stress Anxiety/fear	Depression	Psychological problems	Depression	Depression	Mood swings	Mood swings	Depression Dementia	
PHYSICAL MANIFESTATIONS									
GENERAL AND METABOLIC	Frequent, often un-explained headaches Chronic fatigue Sleep disturbance	Ataxia Chronic fatigue		Fatigue	Headaches Insomnia Fatigue	Fatigue	Headaches	Fatigue	Fatigue (mal-absorption of Vitamin C)

VISION		Decreased eye coordination	Hypersensitivity to light Impaired vision					Inflammation of the optic nerve	
SKIN, NAILS, HAIR, TEETH	A white line appears when skin is scratched Brown spots on face, neck and shoulders		Seborrhoea	Skin problems Erythema	Skin problems Hair loss	Seborrheic Dermatitis Inflammation of the corners of the mouth		Pale face Wounds take a long time to heal	Bleeding gums Wounds take a long time to heal Dental fragility
VASCULAR	Sensitivity to cold Hypotension Dizziness Loss of consciousness Arrhythmia/palpitations Shortness of breath	Hypertrophy and heart failure		Haematological problems Regulates cholesterol			Palpitations	Palpitations	
IMMUNE	Swollen lymph nodes (in the neck or neck glands) Associated with auto-immune diseases Catches colds easily		Inflammation of mucus membrane		Respiratory inflections Immune deficiency				
INTESTINAL	Digestive problems Weight loss Salt cravings	Nausea Loss of appetite Constipation		Swollen tongue Loss of appetite Diarrhoea	Nausea Abdominal pain Diarrhoea	Swollen tongue Digestive problems Malabsorption Weight loss	Swollen tongue Loss of appetite Weight loss Change in mucosal cells Diarrhoea	Swollen tongue Loss of appetite Weight loss Flatulence Constipation	Digestive problems Malabsorption Weight loss

	ADRENAL FATIGUE	THIAMINE B1 DEFICIENCY	RIBOFLAVIN B2 DEFICIENCY	NIACIN NICOTINAMIDE B3 DEFICIENCY	PENTATONIC ACID B5 DEFICIENCY	PYRIDOXINE B6 DEFICIENCY	FOLIC ACID B9 DEFICIENCY	CYANOCOBALAMIN B12 DEFICIENCY	VITAMIN C DEFICIENCY
REPRODUCTIVE AND URINARY	Enhanced PMS (10 days) Decreased sexual desire						Change in mucosal cells		
MUSCULO-SKELETAL	Tremors: *When stressed* Swollen ankles at night Agitated arms and legs Muscle weakness	Cramps Muscle weakness	Tingling in the hands and feet Lack of stability when standing	Weakness	Paraesthesia of the limbs Tingling, burning sensation or numbness Cramps			Tingling and numbness Numbness Burning sensation in the limbs Weakness	Oedema Joint pain Muscular fatigue Cartilage and muscle degeneration
OTHER ASSOCIATED CONDITIONS	Allergies Multiple chemical sensitivities Respiratory diseases Rheumatoid arthritis Fibromyalgia Other immune and auto-immune diseases	Wernicke-Korsakoff syndrome		Psycho-logical problems Pellagra Hartnup's disease	Anaemia Hypo-glycaemia	Sideroblastic anaemia	Megaloblastic anaemia Growth delay	Anaemia	Anaemia Scurvy

Appendix 2C: Nutritional Deficiencies – Fat-Soluble Vitamins

	SYMPTOMS OF ADRENAL FATIGUE	BETA-CAROTENE VITAMIN A	CALCITRIOL VITAMIN D	TOCOPHEROLS VITAMIN E	VITAMIN K MENAQUINONE MENADIONE PHYLLOQUINONE
COGNITIVE AND EMOTIONAL MANIFESTATIONS					
COGNITIVE	Trouble concentrating Forgetfulness Decreased mental clarity Irritability Decreased productivity Mental confusion when in a hurry			Poor nerve conduction	
EMOTIONAL	Inability to tolerate stress Feelings of despair Anxiety/fear				
PHYSICAL MANIFESTATIONS					
GENERAL AND METABOLIC	Chronic headaches Frequent, often unexplained Sleep disorder Sudden drops in energy Chronic fatigue	Headaches Mucosal dryness (lungs)		Lipid metabolism disturbance	
VISION		Night blindness Xerophtalmia Conjunctivitis		Retina abnormalities	

	SYMPTOMS OF ADRENAL FATIGUE	BETA-CAROTENE VITAMIN A	CALCITRIOL VITAMIN D	TOCOPHEROLS VITAMIN E	VITAMIN K MENAQUINONE MENADIONE PHYLLOQUINONE
SKIN, NAILS, HAIRS	A white line appears when skin is scratched Brown spots appear on the face, neck and shoulders	Dry skin Premature ageing of the skin Dandruff Hair loss			
VASCULAR	Hypotension Dizziness Fainting Arrhythmia/palpitations Shortness of breath		Coronary diseases	Capillary fragility	Blood coagulation failure
PHYSICAL MANIFESTATIONS					
IMMUNE	Swollen lymph nodes (neck and arm pits) Associated with auto-immune diseases Catches colds easily	Decreased tolerance to infections			
GASTRO-INTESTINAL	Weight loss Poor digestion Salt cravings	Mucosal dryness Nausea Abdominal pain Diarrhoea Loss of appetite		Malabsorption	Malabsorption
REPRODUCTIVE AND URINARY	Exacerbated PMS (10 days) Decreased sexual desire	Mucosal dryness			
MUSCULOSKELETAL	Tremors: *When stressed* Swollen ankles at night Agitated limbs	*Impaired bone mineralization* Muscle and joint pain	Bone pain Muscle weakness	Myopathy	

OTHER ASSOCIATED CONDITIONS	Allergies Multiple chemical sensitivities Respiratory diseases Rheumatoid arthritis Fibromyalgia Other immune and auto-immune disease	Allergies Skin disease Osteoporosis	Multiple sclerosis Fibromyalgia Osteomalacia Rickets Cancer, Type II diabetes	Anaemia due to fewer red blood cells	Osteoporosis

References

Michael W. King, 'The medical biochemistry page,' National Science Teachers Association, http://themedicalbiochemistrypage.org.

Vulgaris Médical, 'Vitamin B2,' www.vulgaris-medical.com/front/?p=index_fiche&id_article=4817.

Medline Plus, 'Vitamin A,' www.nlm.nih.gov/medlineplus/ency/article/002400.htm#References.

Vulgaris Médical. 'Acide pantothenique,' www.vulgaris-medical.com/front/?p=index_fiche&id_article=139.

Passeport santé, www.passeportsante.net/fr/Solutions/PlantesSupplements/Index.aspx.

Pitchford Paul, *Healing with Whole Foods*, Berkeley, North Atlantic Books, 2002.

Office of Dietary Supplements, National Institute of Health, http://dietary-supplements.info.nih.gov/Health_Information/Vitamin_and_Mineral_Supplement_Fact_Sheets.aspx.

Appendix 3: Environmental Stressors

In occupational therapy we evaluate the occupational performance of the person in his environment, based on three categories: physical, social, and cultural. Is it dangerous? Are there new elements that can explain what is happening with the client? Is it safe to return to this environment? Should it be adapted to the client's needs? As a last resort, should it be completely changed in order to optimize the individual's functional reintegration into his environment? The following list is an overview of the possible stressors from the exhausted person's physical environment that could potentially have an energy-draining effect on his condition. Almost all the physical stimuli are listed based on the senses, which helps bodily messages to be more easily decoded when we are exposed to such stimuli. In the same way that one stressor may be experienced in different ways, it may be repeated more than once. Of these stressors, some can be partially and others totally eliminated to restore the PNI balance in people who have been battling them.

Are you *frequently* exposed or have you been frequently exposed to one or more of the following stressors?

Computer screen (many hours per day)

TV (many hours per day)

Wi-Fi, cellular phone use (more than 15 minutes/day)

Relay antenna for cellular phone technology
(more than 0.2V/m in home environment)

Screen watching with rapid image change
(video clip, publicity movies…)

Reading documents over many consecutive hours

Lack of darkness at night

Loud music (bar, house, work environment…)

Big city background noise

Construction site

Antibacterial soap

Commercial hair dye

Tattoos

Ink: printer, newspaper

Smog averaging 1 day out of 7, meaning living
or working in a big city on a regular basis

First-hand or second-hand smoking

Tar: roofing, asphalt, underlay

Exhaust fumes (work in a garage, a car park...)

Oil or gas heating (including fireplace and stove)

Synthetic perfumes: own or in surroundings at work (beauty
parlour, cosmetics section in stores, fashion industry...)

Petroleum derivatives: gas, candles, skin cream, soft plastic,
especially in a warm environment (microwave oven, next
to a furnace or welding tools...), synthetic clothing

Synthetic antiperspirant and deodorant

Chemical vapours: hairspray, oven spray, detergents
(chlorhydric, sulphuric, or phosphoric acid), etc.

Moulds (damp basement, air conditioned office building...)

Dust (especially near highways, wood or plaster dust)

Cleaning products (containing phosphate,
concentrated javex, oven cleaner ammonium)

Pollen

Rubber, asbestos, paint, solvents, adhesive, formaldehyde

Heavy metals: living in a house that is more
than 50 years old, old dental amalgams

Refined sugar

Trans fat

Food colouring (derived or petroleum-based) and additives

Flavour enhancers (MSG)

Synthetic sweeteners (saccharine, aspartame), refined flour

Stimulants: caffeine, guarana, chocolate, etc.

Untreated cavities, old dental amalgams

Pesticides, insecticides, fungicides (xeno-oestrogens)

Appendix 4: Energy Balance Sheet

DIMENSIONS		PHYSICAL		EMOTIONAL		COGNITIVE		SOCIOCULTURAL		SPIRITUAL	
CATEGORIES	ACTIVITIES	SYMPA-THETIC	PARASYM-PATHETIC	FEAR	COURAGE	DUTY	PLEASURE	OTHERS	SELF	POWERLESS-NESS	POWER
REST											
	Night										
	Nap										
	Health break										
PERSONAL HYGIENE											
	Dressing/undressing										
	Washing										
	Grooming										
PRODUCTIVITY											
ACTIVITIES OF DAILY LIVING (ADL)	Groceries										
	Washing dishes										
	House repair										
	Organizing finances										
	Taking care of pets										

WORK												
	Paid work											
	Volunteer work											
	Care to relatives, friends											
	Care to children											
LEISURE												
	Social activities											
	Gardening											
	Reading											
	Sport											
TOTAL %	NUMBERS OF HOURS 'X' OR '%'											

Inspired by C. A. Trombly, *Occupational Therapy for Physical Dysfunction* (2nd edition), Baltimore, Williams & Wilkins, 1983; Association canadienne des ergothérapeutes, *Lignes directrices pour une pratique de l'ergothérapie centrée sur le client*, Toronto, Publications ACE, 1993; and M. Law *et al. La Mesure canadienne du rendement occupationnel*, Ottawa, Publications ACE, 1994.

- The left-hand column of each dimension is at the *energy-draining* polarity and the right-hand column is at the *energizing* polarity.
- Enter an X for each of the dimensions of your selected activities based on the instructions provided in the sections of Chapter 4.
- It is possible to check two polarities for the same dimension.
- If you prefer, use percentages.
- Complete your energy balance sheet while calculating the total of your selections per column or by calculating the average of the percentages based on what concerns you the most or the number of X per category.
- Do this for each of the dimensions and make a note of your observations.

Appendix 5: Daily Energy Scale

SCALE	%	ACTIVE HOURS	DEFINITION	METS
5	100%	16 & more	Over and above the daily demands of work, can physically train with intensity without experiencing a return of symptoms	9 & more
4.5	97.5%	16 & more	When at 95%, can physically train with intensity on a non-work day without experiencing a return of symptoms but not on a work day	9 & more
4	95%	16 & more	Performs all daily activities and occupations with sustained intensity without difficulty and without experiencing a return of symptoms	7 to 8
3.5	92.5%	16 & more	Performs all daily activities and occupations with rest periods (may experience a return of fatigue or abnormal pain)	7 to 8
3	90%	16 & more	Full day at work (productive day and evening) without energy decrease for 7 days (stability of energy level despite the increased effort)	6 to 7
2.5	87.5%	16 & more	Full day at work (productive day and evening) without energy decrease for 7 days (fatigue or abnormal pain present)	6 to 7
2	85%	16 & more	7-hour day of work (2 periods of 3 hours and 30 min) (returned to part-time work)	6 to 7
1.5	82.5%	16 & more	7-hour day of work (2 periods of 3 hours and 30 min) (fatigue or abnormal pain present)	6 to 7
1	80%	16 & more	Demanding half days without marked decrease in energy for 3 consecutive days (no signs of fatigue or abnormal pain)	6 to 7
0.5	77.5%	16 & more	Demanding half days without marked decrease in energy for 3 consecutive days (fatigue or abnormal pain present)	6 to 7
0	75%	16 & more	Works 3 consecutive hours (physical or mental) with sustained intensity (returned to part-time work)	6 to 7
-0.5	72.5%	16 & more	Works 3 consecutive hours (physical or mental) with sustained intensity (fatigue or abnormal pain present)	6 to 7
-1	70%	16 & more	Performs daily routine with some physical or mental demands (has energy during the evening)	5 to 6
-1.5	67.5%	16 & more	Performs daily routine with some physical or mental demands (demanding activity followed by fatigue or abnormal pain)	5 to 6
-2	65%	16 & more	Performs daily activities – except sustained physical or mental activities	4 to 5
-2.5	62.5%		Remove 0.5 if needs at least a 30-minute rest	4 to 5
-3	60%	15 to 16	Day without major stressors but decreased energy the next day	3 to 4
-3.5	57.5%		Remove 0.5 if needs at least a 30-minute rest	3 to 4
-4	55%	15	Needs a nap or a rest (nap time is not included in the active time)	3 to 4

-4.5	52.5%	Remove 0.5 if needs at least a 30-minute rest		3 to 4
-5	50%	Needs a nap or a rest (nap time is not included in the active time)	14	3 to 4
-5.5	47.5%	Remove 0.5 if needs at least a 30-minute rest		3 to 4
-6	45%	Needs a nap or a rest (nap time is not included in the active time)	13	3 to 4
-6.5	42.5%	Remove 0.5 if needs at least a 30-minute rest		3 to 4
-7	40%	Needs a nap in the afternoon and other rest periods during the day	12	3 to 4
-7.5	37.5%	Remove 0.5 if needs at least a 30-minute rest (nap time is not included in the active time)		3 to 4
-8	35%	Needs a nap and a rest during the day (nap time is not included in the active time)	11	3 to 4
-8.5	32.5%	Remove 0.5 at least a 30-minute rest		3 to 4
-9	30%	Needs to sleep during the day during between more demanding instrumental activities of daily living (making a meal, doing laundry...)	10	3 to 4
-10	27.5%	Needs to sleep during the day between basic self-care activities	9	3 to 4
-11	25%	Needs to sleep during the day between basic self-care activities	8	3 to 4
-12	22.5%	Can prepare simple meals, has to sit often, needs a nap and goes to bed early	7	2 to 3
-13	20%	Energy in the morning and around 6:00 pm only, in bed or sitting for the remainder of the time	6	2 to 3
-14	17.5%	Energy in the morning at around 10:00 am or in the evening only, in bed for the remainder of the time	5	2 to 3
-15	15%	A bit of energy, most likely in the late morning or at around supper time	4	2 to 3
-16	12.5%	In bed or sitting, can do basic self-care activities	3	2 to 3
-17	10%	In bed, except to eat and go to the bathroom	2	1.5 to 2
-18	5%	In bed, may be able to go to the bathroom	1	1

Abnormal fatigue is defined in the DES as sudden fatigue that follows a physical or mental effort or after feeling stressed or emotional. It can also be considered abnormal when present in the morning even after a good night's sleep or if fatigue comes on suddenly at certain times during the day (e.g. around 11:00 am and 4:00 pm).

Abnormal pain is defined as a disproportionate muscle or joint pain in relation to the level of physical activity performed or even in the absence of any physical activity. It can also be diffused pain of unknown origin, non-specific to muscles or joints and present at all times.

For insomniacs: Calculate *active hours* as being the hours in which you are out of bed (24 hours less the hours spent in bed, even if you don't sleep).

Appendix 6: Cognitive Scale

The problem with assessing cognitive symptoms is that they may appear at different points during the day and disappear a few hours later.

It is preferable to assess yourself at the end of the day in order to have an overall picture of your performance.

SCALE	DEFINITION
0	Functional
-1	Suffers from a slight decrease in mental sharpness (mental fatigue) Has mild organizational problems (unusually sloppy; creates messes)
-2	Has a slight decrease in his ability to think rationally (especially in response to stress)
-3	Has trouble concentrating after a meal or after physical exertion, mildly impaired in making decisions
-4	Irritable, intolerant to noise, can do continuous intellectual work for at least two hours except during the evening
-5	Forgetful, has difficulty finding words, frequently indecisive, has to take notes not to forget
-6	Has obvious organizational problems, is frequently forgetful (leaves cupboard doors open, disorganized with paperwork, bills to pay, food in the refrigerator, etc.)
-7	Attention span moderately impaired by too many environmental stimuli (music, children, noise) Has a difficult time multitasking (driving while listening to the radio) Frequently indecisive
-8	Attention span is severely impaired by too many outside stimuli (music, odours, noise) even when doing only one thing at a time Cannot read (no concentration), cannot meditate (mind constantly wanders)
-9	Cannot drive a car, cannot concentrate on someone else talking, constantly indecisive
-10	Suffers from thought perseveration (as if an idea or a sentence was constantly repeating itself in a loop with no end in sight) or perseveration in body movements (automatic repetitive gestures)

Appendix 7: Psychomotor Agitation Scale

SCALE	DEFINITION
4	Severe psychomotor agitation Insomnia, spasms at night (when going to bed, during the night or both) Constant irritability, feels edgy all the time Paralysing perfectionism, severe difficulty in making decisions Severe disorganization, searching for words, constant forgetfulness
3	Moderate psychomotor agitation, exhausted at night. Eyes wide open in a *fight or flight* mode Often wakes up at night for one or two hours, seeks stimulants in the morning (caffeine) Irritability in the late morning and in the late afternoon, very emotional Constantly dissatisfied with others' work, no longer delegates work Trouble concentrating at night, forgetful, disorganized
2	Mild psychomotor agitation, full of energy, a bit hyperactive but performs at a high level Mild sleep disturbance, difficulty waking up in the morning, drawn to alcohol or sedatives at the end of the day to slow down Weekend irritability (Friday), more emotional than usual Perfectionist, impatient, finishes sentences for others, disappointed by others Mild attention difficulty, extreme verbal fluidity
1	Performs highly, can multitask easily Highly functional on little sleep, hypervigilant during the day Occasionally irritable Very sharp and alert Hyperefficient at work, feels very lucid
0	Normal

Appendix 8A: Monthly Energy Time Sheet

Monthly fluctuation of energy level

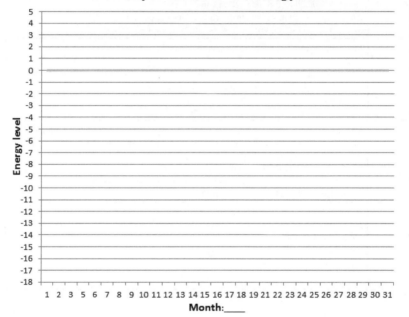

Appendix 8B: Monthly Data (Cognitive Abilities)

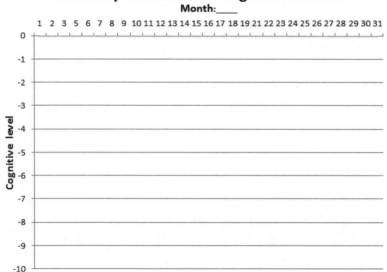

Monthly fluctuation of cognitive abilities
Month:____

Appendix 8C: Monthly Data (Psychomotor Agitation)

Monthly fluctuation of cognitive abilities

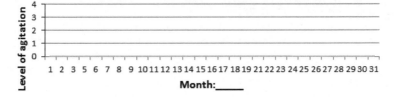

Appendix 9A: Beneficial Effects of Dietary Supplements – Vitamins

DIRECT OR INDIRECT EFFECT (COFACTOR, ETC.)	VITAMINS											
	A	B1	B2	B3	B5	B6	B9	B12	C	D	E	K
MENTAL												
Beneficial effect								x				
Myelin synthesis								x				
EMOTIONAL												
Necessary for neurotransmitter production				x		x			x			
Nervous system functioning							x					
Calming effect												
METABOLIC												
DNA and/or RNA synthesis						x	x	x	x		x	
Amino acids			x						x			
Catabolism of fatty acids								x				
Energy production-ATP (mitochondria)		x	x	x	x	x		x	x			
Antioxidants	x								x		x	
Maintenance of connective tissue									x			
Protection of mucous membranes										x		
HORMONAL												
Calcitonin and parathyroid hormone functions										x		
Adrenal hormone manufacturing cascade		x	x	x	x	x	x	x	x		x	
Adrenal gland metabolism						x			x			
Help maintain a normal blood glucose level				x		x		x	x			
Necessary for sexual hormone production						x						
Necessary for cholesterol metabolism					x							
Strengthening cellular membrane	x											

DIRECT OR INDIRECT EFFECT (COFACTOR, ETC.)	VITAMINS											
	A	B1	B2	B3	B5	B6	B9	B12	C	D	E	K
VISION Protection against night blindness	x											
Beneficial effect on cataracts										x		
SKIN Beneficial effects	x				x				x			
NAILS, BONES Beneficial effects										x		
HAIR Beneficial effects												
VASCULAR Decreases blood clotting											x	
Protection									x			
Red blood cell formation						x	x	x				
Haemoglobin formation				x		x	x					
Normal blood clotting												x
Regulates blood cholesterol level					x							
IMMUNE Promotes a healthy immune system	x					x	x		x	x		
INTESTINAL Control synthesis of bile salts									x			
Positive effect, decreases risk of inflammation								x				
Absorption of iron and chrome									x			
Absorption of phosphorus and calcium										x		

Appendix 9B: Beneficial Effects of Dietary Supplements – Minerals and Others

DIRECT OR INDIRECT EFFECT (COFACTOR, ETC.)	MINERALS								OTHERS	
	Mg	Ca	Fe	K	Cr	Mn	Se	Zn	CoQ10	Omega-3
MENTAL										
Nervous system functioning			x	x						x
Calming effect	x	x	x	x		x	x	x		x
METABOLIC										
DNA and/or RNA synthesis							x	x		
Cellular growth			x							
Energy production-ATP (mitochondria)	x		x						x	
Sense of smell								x		
Calcium metabolism	x									
Stimulate vitamin B group										
Antioxidants						x	x	x	x	
HORMONAL										
Adrenal hormone manufacturing cascade	x									
Adrenal gland metabolism	x			x				x		
Regulate the action of insulin					x					x
Effect of carbohydrate, protein and fat metabolism				x	x					
Required for thyroid hormone synthesis							x			
Decrease PMS symptoms	x									x

	DIRECT OR INDIRECT EFFECT (COFACTOR, ETC.)	MINERALS								OTHERS	
		Mg	Ca	Fe	K	Cr	Mn	Se	Zn	CoQ10	Omega-3
URINARY	Kidney regeneration	x									
	Kidney stone prevention				x						
	Anti-inflammatory effect on prostate	x									
SKIN, NAILS, BONES, HAIR	Beneficial effect	x					x				
	Bone, teeth, nails, and hair restoration	x	x								
VASCULAR	Decreases blood clotting										x
	Promotes blood clotting				x						
	Prevention of hypertension	x	x		x					x	x
	Prevention of tachycardia	x									
	Prevention of arrhythmia	x			x						
	Protective effect		x							x	x
	Necessary for oxygen transportation in the blood stream			x							
	Reduces blood cholesterol	x									
	Increases good cholesterol (HDL)					x					x
IMMUNE	Sustain proper immune functions								x		
	Anti-allergenic	x		x			x				
	Anti-inflammatory	x					x	x			x
	Bactericide	x									

INTESTINAL	Calming effect on the stomach	x	
	Regenerative effect on the liver	x	
	Positive effect on digestion	x	
	Positive effect on Ca, P, Na, and K absorption	x	
	Repair of intestinal wall	x	x
MUSCULO-SKELETAL	Muscle relaxation	x	
	Muscle contraction	x	

References

Michael W. King, 'The medical biochemistry page,' http://themedicalbiochemistrypage.org.
www.vulgaris-medical.com/encyclopedie.html.
Medline Plus, 'Vitamine A,' www.nlm.nih.gov/medlineplus/ency/article/002400.htm#References.
Passeport santé, www.passeportsante.net/fr/Solutions/PlantesSupplements/Index.aspx.
www.courir.org/biosante/biosante_magnesium.html.
Office of Dietary Supplements, http://ods.od.nih.gov/Health_Information/Information_About_Individual_Dietary_Supplements.aspx.
Paul Pitchford, *Healing with Whole Foods*, Berkeley, North Atlantic Books, 2002.
Alan R. Gaby, *The Natural Pharmacy* (3rd edition), New York, Three Rivers Press, 2006.

Glossary

Adjustment disorder: Group of symptoms linked to stress and caused by one or more overwhelming stressors in relation to the person's ability to face it. By definition, according to the medical field, it lasts at most six months.

Adrenal: Related to the endocrine glands located above the kidneys and involved in body–mind reactions to stress.

Adrenocorticotropic hormone (ACTH): Also known as corticotropin. Produced and secreted by the anterior pituitary gland, it stimulates the adrenal cortex to release corticosteroids.

Aerobic: Related to an environment dependent on oxygen to live.

Anaerobic: Related to an environment in which life can develop in the absence of oxygen.

Androgen: Steroid hormone that promotes the development of male sexual organs and male secondary sexual characteristics.

Autonomic nervous system (ANS): Also known as the neurovegetative system or vegetative system, this is the part of the nervous system that regulates key functions (breathing, blood circulation, digestion, excretion) in the body through control of the smooth muscles, the heart muscle, and the glands. The ANS has two divisions, the sympathetic and the parasympathetic nervous systems.

Brainstem: Lower extension of the brain formed by the medulla oblongata, midbrain and pons. It is part of the reptilian brain where survival and arousal functions and ANS rhythms are controlled (breathing, cardiac, sleep rhythms, etc.).

Bruxism: Involuntary clenching or grinding of the teeth during sleep.

Burn-out: Gradual physical and emotional exhaustion, due to perceived stress from working under demanding and/or difficult conditions. It is not a medical diagnosis. It will come as a diagnosis of an adjustment disorder if it lasts a maximum of six months.

Chronobiology: The study of the effects of time and rhythmic phenomena on life processes.

Circadian rhythm: Biological cycle of active and non-active periods in an organism. It is determined by internal physical, mental, and behavioural changes that roughly follow a 24-hour cycle encompassing sleep, hormonal, and secretion patterns.

Clock time: Chronological concept of time: past, present, and future. It allows us to take into account past experiences and plan the future in order to fully live in the present.

Cortisol: The hormone secreted by the medulla of the adrenal glands, with anti-inflammatory and hyperglycemic effects, among others. This hormone is considered the 'stress hormone'.

Courage: In the present context, courage is defined as the will to confront change. It is a feeling that allows us to face life changes and challenges.

Cranial nerve: There are 12 pairs of cranial nerves emerging from the brain and the brain stem compared to our 31 pairs of spinal nerves related to the spinal cord.

Dogma: A corpus of doctrine set forth as a fundamental truth that cannot be questioned.

Ego or self: In psychoanalysis, the ego is one of the three divisions of the psyche that plays the role of mediator between the instincts of the *id* and the critical and moralizing *super-ego*. In this book, we specify that the ego is an image we have of ourselves, modelled by our conditioning, and that allows us to deal with daily reality.

Emotion: Psychological response that manifests itself mainly as autonomic nervous system activity.

Energy: Commonly defined as a physical system's capacity to do work, such as producing heat, light or movement. It can be regarded as the common currency or information that can be exchanged during physical phenomena. The information would therefore be the energy that is first perceived by our senses and subsequently transferred inside of us.

Exteroceptor: Sensory cell that receives information from outside the body.

Fear: Emotion felt when faced with danger, pain, etc.

Force: In the present context, force is defined as a survival reaction, observed as aggressive and opposing, as a result of a skewed perception of being vulnerable or isolated.

Glucose: The body's major energy source.

Glycogen: Main form of carbohydrate storage in the body.

Glycogenesis: The formation of glycogen from glucose for storage in the liver.

Glycogenolysis: The biochemical breakdown of glycogen into glucose.

Glycolysis: The intracellular process of breaking down glucose to produce energy (ATP). It is the metabolic pathway that increases energy release by way of carbohydrate oxidation. It converts glucose into lactic acid in an anaerobic environment and pyruvate in aerobic glycolysis. This conversion is strictly reserved for carbohydrates. All 11 reactions of the aerobic glycolysis require different catalysts (enzymes) from which water and carbon dioxide are produced as waste.

Glycemic index: A scale that ranks carbohydrates on a scale of 10 to 110 where *glucose* ranks 100. It describes the capacity of different foods containing carbohydrates to stimulate the production of the hormone insulin.

Homeostasis: The ability of the organism or cell to regulate its internal physiological dynamic balance of the body such as inner temperature, pH, oxygen level, regardless of the external changing conditions.

Hippocampus: Component of the brain that plays a major role in working memory commonly known as short-term memory.

Hyperglycemias: Excessive level of glucose in the blood.

Hypoglycaemia: A lower-than-normal level of blood glucose.

Info-energy: Information on the environment that reaches our body–mind from our senses through chemical, electrical, and possibly magnetic paths, reaching all the cells of our super PNI system. For example, regardless of whether this information is visual or auditory, it is an energy signal that our body–mind picks up, decodes then transmits, hence the name info-energy.

Information: A concept that allows the transfer, storage, and process of knowledge. We draw the analogy between information and energy because emission, reception, and retransmission of the energy as signals or a combination of signals need to be picked up as information by our senses to reach our body–mind.

Insulin: Hormone secreted by the pancreas that controls the blood glucose level by allowing the glucose to enter cells, therefore it has a hypoglycaemic effect.

Learned helplessness: Psychological term developed by Dr Martin Seligman while he was conducting animal studies and the effect of electric shocks on their behaviour: apathy and learned helplessness were observed. The concept, extended to human behaviour, can take place when people feel that they cannot have an impact on their environment and that they cannot change the situation they are facing to work in their favour.

Leaky gut syndrome: A condition in which the intestinal permeability has been altered, thereby allowing large molecules to penetrate the body whereas in normal conditions they would not. This increased porosity is caused by antibiotics, toxins, poor diet parasites, or infection and therefore inflammation. Alcohol and spice consumption can further increase the pathogenic permeability and perpetuate the vicious cycle, leading to further inflammation and resulting in immune system dysfunction.

Long-term memory: This memory allows us to encode, store, and retrieve information in an organized manner.

Malabsorption syndrome: Difficulty digesting or absorbing nutrients (carbohydrates lipids, proteins) associated with intestinal wall damage. This type of condition can lead to an abnormal loss of weight, oedema in the lower extremities, anemia, chronic diarrhoea, and metabolic diseases.

Metabolic equivalent (MET): A way of measuring the energy cost of physical activities. It specifically measures the quantity of oxygen required per minute to perform a physical task: 1 MET = 3.5 ml oxygen/min/kg of body weight. 1 MET is the energy required to maintain *homeostasis*, or all the organ functions of the body at rest. Between 3 and 6 METS, activities are considered to be of moderate intensity. Above 6 METS, the intensity is considered vigourous. In Chapter 5, there is a list of activities with their energy expenditure estimate in METS.

Neurotransmitters: Also known as neuromediators, these are a variety of synthesized molecules with axonal endings (*axon*: long process of nerve fibres). Playing the role of chemical messengers, neurotransmitters are released in response to a potential action by nervous cells.

Neuropeptide: Neurotransmitter and peptide.

Neurovegetative: Group of nerve structures that controls major involuntary functions: circulation, secretion, excretion, etc.

Paradigm: A pattern or model.

Peptide: A group of compounds formed by two or more amino acids linked by a carboxyl group of others, or by hydrolysis of proteins. Many peptides act as info-energy messengers in our body. We call them neuropeptides or neurotransmitters because they are released in the brain. However, it is now a scientific fact that many of them can be produced in other organs.

Peristaltism or peristalsis: Intestinal wavy reflex movement. This movement is controled by the parasympathetic branch of the ANS and starts in the oesophagus and propagates in a rhythmic fashion to the anus. That wave propagation is triggered by the food present in the digestive tube.

Photon emission: Electromagnetic energy that radiates from any life system that is caused by its metabolic activity.

Photosynthesis: The process in green plants and certain other organisms by which carbon dioxide and water, using sunlight as an energy source, can synthesize carbohydrates.

Pleasure: In this book pleasure is related to the neurochemical response of the pleasure centre in the brain during a given activity or situation. This response is broader than the hedonistic enjoyment through the senses. The response from the pleasure centre is elicited by the satisfaction associated with the activity from which we derive a sustained interest or by the fact that we are engaging in an activity with a playful attitude. It can also be defined as the positive perception that results from the interest we have in an activity, from the way we perform that activity or from the attitude we have during that activity.

Power: In this book we consider power to be the self-assertiveness in harmony with one's deep life convictions in relation to the environment and, for some people, with respect to their connection with the universe.

Psychological time: A perception of time that is not reality and that we superimpose onto *clock time*. Psychological time projects us into the future or makes us return to the past and prevents us from living in the present moment.

Psycho-neuro-immuno-endocrine (PNI) system: According to the emerging scientific paradigm, it is the concept of the super system in which all the different systems of the body are constantly interacting with one another and influence each other in a more fluid way than was believed at the end of the twentieth century. In previous centuries, science used a reductionist model to understand the body–mind. This new super model was introduced close to 30 years ago to better illustrate the interactions between all the body systems.

Serotonin: A chemical messenger involved, among other things, in nutritional and sexual behaviour, the sleep cycle, aggressiveness, pain, and depression.

Short-term memory: A 'buffer' memory also called *working memory*. It allows us to temporarily hold on to a piece of information. We do not necessarily remember the data we worked with at that level.

Sleep apnoea: Temporary stoppage of breathing during sleep (apnoea) or shallow breathing periods (hypopnoea) during sleep. It is associated with periods of persistent fatigue and sleepiness during the day.

Stress: Non-specific reaction of the organism that requires an adjustment or adaptation. This adaptation can be triggered by physiological factors (taking a hot bath, breathing at high altitudes, engaging in exercise, etc.) or psychological (pleasant or not) factors (eating acidic foods, being exposed to pollution, etc.). For Hans Selye, these reactions are non-specific and cannot be avoided.

Syndrome: A set of symptoms that characterize a disease or a disorder.

Thymus: Immune system gland that secretes peptides that will then bring T-cells (T for thymus) – also called T-lymphocytes – into maturation.

Working memory: Short-term memory.

Endnotes

Introduction

1. An *adjustment disorder* is a group of symptoms lasting less than six months reflecting a failure to adapt to one or more overwhelming stressors. The more stressors there are, the more difficult it is to adapt to changes that occur, during a war or Hurricane Katrina, for example. We will come back to this in Chapter 1.
2. Bernie S. Siegel, *Love, Medicine and Miracles*, New York, Harper & Row, 1986, pp.18–26.

How to Use this Book

1. Matthew 7.7–7.8.

Chapter 1

1. To gain a sense of the validity and reliability of the instrument, see M. Horowitz *et al.* 'Life event questionnaires for measuring presumptive stress,' *Psychosomatic Medicine*, vol. 39, no. 6, Nov–Dec 1977.
2. Reprinted from H. Holmes and R. H. Rahe, 'The social readjustment rating scale,' *Journal of Psychosomatic Research*, vol 11(2), August 1967, p.214, with permission from Elsevier.
3. Some medication can also cause the symptoms listed. Also, while you are doing this exercise, make a list of the different medication that you take, prescribed or not. This will be useful for you and for the professionals who will work with you in your process.
4. David Servan-Schreiber, *Guérir: le stress, l'anxiété et la dépression sans médicaments ni psychanalyse*, Paris, Robert Laffont, 2003, p.18.
5. Expression used by the physiologist Bradford Cannon.
6. Hans Selye, *The Stress of Life*, New York, McGraw-Hill Paperbacks, 1956, p.65.
7. Here is a good example of the impact on the psycho-neuro-immuno-endocrine system.
8. Here are three different authors who try to understand the disease and to eliminate the causes rather than the symptoms: W. H. Philpott and D. K. Kalita, *Brain Allergies* (second edition), Chicago, Keats Publishing, 2000; T. Randolph and R. Moss, *An Alternative Approach to Allergies* (revised edition), New York, Harper and Row Publishers, 1990; Janine Fontaine, *Les Maux méprisés*, Paris, Robert Laffont, 1992.
9. J. Wass and S. Shalet, *Oxford Textbook of Endocrinology and Diabetes*, Bath, Oxford University Press, 2002.
10. James L. Wilson, *Adrenal Fatigue: The 21st Century Stress Syndrome*, Petaluma, CA, Smart Publications, 2001, p.49.
11. Conference paper by Dr John Stewart, neurologist, 'Orthostatic hypotension: under diagnosed and under-treated?' Montreal Neurological Institute, 2002.
12. Karl Kraus (1874–1936), Trans. by Harry Zohn, *Half-Truths and One-and-a-Half Truths*, Chicago, University of Chicago Press, 1990 (originally published in Beim Wort genommen, 1955).

13. Dr Jacob Teitelbaum, Online question and answer sessions, FM-CFS Canada, www.fm-cfs.ca/ QATeitelbaum.html; James L. Wilson, *Adrenal Fatigue: The 21st Century Stress Syndrome*, Petaluma, CA, Smart Publications, 2001.

14. A.D. Sperber *et al*. 'Fibromyalgia in the irritable bowel syndrome: studies of prevalence and clinical implications,' *Am J Gastroenterol*, Dec 1999, 94(12): 3541–3546; H. Mertz., V. Morgan., G. Tanner *et al*. 'Regional cerebral activation in irritable bowel syndrome,' *Gastroenterology*, 2000, 118: 842–848.

15. Hans Selye, *The Stress of Life*, New York, McGraw-Hill Paperbacks, 1956, pp.31–33.

16. Selye, ibid., p.185.

17. Selye, ibid., p.185.

18. L. Weibell, 'Recommandations méthodologiques préalables à l'utilisation du cortisol salivaire comme marqueur biologique du stress,' *La Presse médicale*, 2003, vol. 32, no. 18, pp.845–851.

19. Each specialized laboratory has its own standards because a medical consensus has not yet been reached for these saliva hormone tests. For this reason, they are used in research, but have not yet been made available by treating physicians.

20. James L. Wilson, *Adrenal Fatigue: The 21st Century Stress Syndrome*, Petaluma, CA, Smart Publications, 2001.

Chapter 2

1.   E.H. Robinson, B.A. Leczynski, F.W. Kutz, J.C. Remmers, 'An evaluation of hexachlorobensene body-burden levels in the general population of the USA,' *IARC Sci Publ*, 1986 (77): 183–193. www.ewg.org/minoritycordblood/BPA-cordbloodpollution

2.   Jean-Marie Pelt and Gilles-Éric Séralini, *Après nous le déluge?* Paris, Flammarion/Fayard, 2006, p.89.

3.   We now know that consuming a spoonful of refined sugar is all that it takes to make the pancreas and adrenal glands work unnecessarily and even paralyse certain cells of the immune system.

4.   To have an idea of the planetary problem of the use of plastic, see the article by Susan Casey available online: 'Plastic ocean,' *Best Life*, Feb 20, 2007, www.raiazome.com/Susan_Casey--Plastic_Ocean

5.   Jean-Marie Pelt and Gilles-Éric Séralini, *Après nous le déluge?* Paris, Flammarion/Fayard, 2006, p.91.

6.   Rick A. Relyea, 'Predator cues and pesticides: a double dose of danger for amphibians,' *Ecological Applications*, 2003, 13(6): 1515–1521.

7.   To learn more about chemicals in our everyday environment and on safer alternatives, visit Safer Products Project: www.safer-products.org

8.   See the video on the International Academy of Medicine and Toxicity website: http://iaomt. org/videos

9.   J. G. Lipson, 'We are the canaries: self-care in multiple chemical sensitivity sufferers,' Department of Community Health Systems, School of Nursing, University of California, San Francisco, USA, *Qual. Health Res*, Jan 2001, 11(1): 103–116.

10. Leakey and Lewin cited by Pelt and Séralini, *Après nous le déluge?* Paris, Flammarion/Fayard, 2006, p.70.

11. Documentary *Doc Monde Épisode: Le paradoxe démographique*, Télé-Québec, 16 April 2007.

12. L. A. Gottschalk, T. Rebello, M. S. Buchsbaum, H. G.Ticker, and E. L. Hodges, 'Abnormalities in hair trace elements as indicators of aberrant behavior,' *Compr Psychiatry*, 1991, May–Jun, 32(2): 229, 37.

13. Carolyne Dean, *The Miracle of Magnesium*, New York, Ballantine Books, 2003, p.28.

14. The Montreal Children's Hospital of the McGill University Health Centre.

15. Eleftherios Zervas *et al*. 'Reduced intracellular Mg concentration in patients with acute asthma,' *Chest*, 2003, 123: 113–118.

16. Andrew L. Stoll, *The Omega-3 Connection*, New York, Simon & Schuster, 2001.

17. David Servan-Schreiber, *Guérir: le stress, l'anxiété et la dépression sans médicaments ni psychanalyse*, Paris, Robert Laffont, 2003, p.147.

18. Servan-Schreiber, ibid.

19. Andrew L. Stoll, *The Omega-3 Connection*, New York, Simon & Schuster, 2001.

20. J. Shulman, *Winning the Food Fight*, Etobicoke, John Wiley & Sons Canada Ltd, 2003; Colette Dumais, naturopath, draws a connection between learning difficulties and the concept of the polluted child. See www.jydionne.com/oligo-elements-et-tdah

21. Larry B. Christensen, *The Food-Mood Connection*, Carrollton, TX: Pro-Health Publications, 1991, p.111.

22. We now know that a mother who has insulin-resistant cells will have a child with the same traits for environmental, not genetic, reasons.

23. Jean-Marie Pelt and Gilles-Éric Séralini, *Après nous le déluge?* Paris, Flammarion/Fayard, 2006; John Lee, J. Hanley and V. Hopkins, *Tout savoir sur la préménopause*, Vannes, Sully, 2001; Catherine Botham, Philip Homes and Paul Harrison, 'Endocrine discruption in mammals, birds, reptiles and amphibians,' *Environmental Science and Technology*, 1999, no. 12; Jane Akre, 'One great big plastic hassle,' Common Ground, March 2007, www.alternet.org/environment/47849/comments/?page=entire

24. Winnie Dunn, 'The sensations of everyday life: empirical, theoretical and pragmatic considerations,' *American Journal of Occupational Therapy*, November/December 2001, vol. 55, no. 6: 608–620; Jean Ayres, *Sensory Integration and Learning Disorders*, Los Angeles, CA, Western Psychological Services, 1972.

25. According to Jeannetta Burpee, an occupational therapist, sensory overload in children is known to lead to a deregulation of physiological and behavioural functions of the central nervous system and especially an imbalance of the ANS functions.

26. Robert Provide, *Le rire, sa vie, son œuvre*, Paris, Robert Laffont, 2003.

27. D. C. McLelland, C. Alexander and E. Marks, 'The need for power, stress, immune function, and illness among male prisoners,' *Journal of Abnormal Psychology*, 1983, 91: 61–70.

28. T. H. Holmes and R. H. Rahe, 'The Social Readjustment Rating Scale,' *Journal of Psychosomatic Research*, 11, 1967: 213–218.

29. Rise in diabetes, depression, and asthma according to Statistics Canada, *Non-transmissible chronic diseases*, www40.statcan.gc.ca/l01/ind01/l3_2966_1887-eng.htm?hili_none; According to Health Canada, 5 per cent of Canadians have claimed to suffer from at least one of three of the following health problems: CFS, fibromyalgia and multiple chemical hypersensitivity. See the study: 'Medically unexplained physical symptoms,' *Health Canada, The Daily*, Friday, January 12 2007, www.statcan.gc.ca/daily-quotidien/070112/dq070112b-eng.htm. Although *professional burnout* is not considered a diagnosis, its prevalence was estimated at 20 per cent in the labour force in 2004; N. Chevrier and S. Renon-Chevrier, 'L'épuisement professionnel: vers des interventions organisationnelles,' *Psychologie Québec*, Nov. 2004.

30. Cited by Candace Pert in *Molecules of Emotion*, New York, Touchstone, 1997, p.305.

31. For further information on Jon Kabat-Zinn and the Mindfulness approach, refer to: www.umassmed.edu/Content.aspx?id=43102

32. All women who I am treating this year who suffer from persistent fatigue and migraines have episodes of migraines when they smell tar.

33. I noted in all my patients who have been suffering from fatigue for a long time, with or without an official diagnosis of myalgic encephalomyelitis, that there was often a history of severe viral infections during childhood: recurring cases of meningitis, Meniere's Disease, cytomegalovirus and gastroenteritis, and middle ear infections. This type of 'co-incidences' supports the not-yet-proven theory stating that one of the multifactorial causes, including a viral infection such as the *Epstein-Barr virus*, may be one of the factors contributing to the syndrome.

Chapter 3

1. Inspired by Mary Law, Sue Baptiste, Anne Carswell-Opzoomer, Mary Ann McColl, Helene Polatajko and Nancy Pollock, *The Canadian Occupational Performance Measure*, Ottawa, Publication CAOT, 1991.

2. David R. Hawkins, *Power versus Force: The Hidden Determinants of Human Behavior*, Carlsbad, Hay House, 2002, p.80.

3.   E. C. Jacobson, *Savoir relaxer*, Montréal: les Éditions de l'homme, 1980, p.59.

4.   David R. Hawkins, *Power versus Force: The Hidden Determinants of Human Behavior*, Carlsbad, Hay House, 2002, p.84.

5.   Martin Seligman, *Learned Optimism: How to Change Your Mind and Your Life*, New York, Vintage, 2006.

6.   Inspired by David R. Hawkins, *Power versus Force: The Hidden Determinants of Human Behavior*, Carlsbad, Hay House, 2002, pp.68–69.

7.   The word 'enthusiasm' comes from the Greek word *enthéos*, which means 'inspired by the gods'. And the gods create the world…through us. *'Obligation'* is derived from the Latin *ob*, meaning 'opposing' and *ligare* 'to relate,' so we are refering to a relationship by constraint. We are far from creativity.

8.   Translated from Serge Mongeau, *La Simplicité volontaire, plus que jamais*, Montréal, Les Éditions Écosociété, 1998, p.173.

9.   Translated from Buzyn Etty, *Papa, maman, laissez-moi le temps de rêver*, Paris, Albin Michel, 1995, p.69.

10.   Employee recognition, *Chair in Occupational Health and Safety Management, Université Laval*, 2006, www.cgsst.com/eng/whats-new-.asp; Louis Trudel and Micheline Saint-Jean, *Réadaptation au travail après un diagnostic d'épuisement professionnel: rôle émergent de l'ergothérapeute.*, CAOT Preconference workshop, May 30, 2006.

11.   Paul Pearsall, *Toxic Success: How to Stop Striving and Start Thriving*, Makawao, Inner Ocean Publishing Inc, 2002.

12.   C. Maslach, 'Burn out: the cost of caring,' *Psychol Health*, 2001, 16(5): 607–611.

13.   Described by Henri Laborit as the behavioural inhibition system (*Système d'inhibition de l'action*), in the 1970s.

14.   E. C. Jacobson, *Savoir relaxer*, Montréal, les Éditions de l'homme, 1980, p.59.

Chapter 4

1.   Paul Pitchford, *Healing with Whole Foods*, Berkeley, North Atlantic Books, 2002, p.78.

2.   C.A. Trombly, *Occupational Therapy for Physical Dysfunction* (2nd edition), Baltimore, Williams & Wilkins, 1983, p.412.

3.   B.E. Ainsworth *et al.* 1993, 'Compendium of physical activities: classification of energy cost of human physical activities,' *Medicine and Science in Sports and Activities*, 1993, 25: 71–80; C.A. Trombly, *Occupational Therapy for Physical Dysfunction* (2nd edition), Baltimore: Williams & Wilkins, 1983; Centers for Disease Control and Prevention, 'Measuring physical activity intensity,' www.cdc.gov/nccdphp/dnpa/physical/measuring/met.htm; Réseau régional de prévention du risque cardio-vasculaire et rénale par l'éducation de patients dépistés, www.reucare.org; The College of Family Physicians of Canada, www.whyiexercise.com/metabolic-equivalent.html

4.   Paul Pitchford, *Healing with Whole Foods*, Berkeley, CA, North Atlantic Books, 2002, p.79.

5.   T. Randolph and R. Moss, *An Alternative Approach to Allergies* (revised edition), New York, Harper and Row, 1990.

6.   If you are interested, I suggest that you refer to the book by T. Randolph and R. Moss, *An Alternative Approach to Allergies* (revised edition), New York, Harper and Row, 1990; Allergy and Environment Health Association Quebec, www.aeha-quebec.ca, accessed December 2011.

7.   For more information on environmental toxicity, consult the following informative website: http://tuberose.com/Environmental_Toxicity.html, accessed December 2011.

8.   I did not include the notion of duration of intensity because in the rehabilitation process truly exhausted people realize that the very fact of increasing the energy demand during a short period of time (2 to 10 minutes) is enough to increase the symptoms.

9.   Although I included a column in percentages, this scale over 100 is not linear, especially for data between 75 and 100 per cent. The scale is adapted for individuals who feel more comfortable with this familiar concept. A scale containing negative data can also be poorly perceived by certain individuals who require all the tangible encouragement possible.

10.   Home Care Services, Quebec Health System, Canada. CLSC stands for Centre local des services communautaires.

Chapter 5

1.   You can find an extensive list in English of alkaline and acidating foods, prepared by Dr Russel Jaffe in 'Food & chemical effects on acid/alkaline body chemical balance,' *Health Studies Collegium*, 2002. Sources include *USDA food data base (Rev 9&10), Food & Nutrition Encyclopedia*; M. Walczak, 'Nutrition applied personally'; H. Aihara, 'Acid & alkaline' see www.google. ca/search?sourceid=navclient&ie=UTF-8&rls=RNWI,RNWI:2005-47,RNWI:en&q=Dr% 2e+Russel+Jaffe%2c+Food+%26+Chemical+Effects+on+Acid%2fAlkaline+Body+Chem ical+Balance+. It is now very clearly documented in medicine that acidity contributes to the inflammatory process and that cancerous cells proliferate in an acid environment.

2.   J. Shulman, *Winning the Food Fight*, Etobicoke, John Wiley & Sons, 2003; James L. Wilson, *Adrenal Fatigue: The 21st Century Stress Syndrome*, Petaluma, CA, Smart Publishing, 2001; Site Biogassendi, http://biogassendi.perso.sfr.fr/indexsuite.htm

3.   Paul Pitchford, *Healing with Whole Foods*, Berkeley, North Atlantic Books, 2002, p.72.

4.   E. J. Vollaard and H. A. Clasener, 'Colonization resistance,' *Antimicrobial Agents and Chemotherapy*, 1994, 38, 409–414.

5.   I have to specify that this chapter is outside my area of professional expertise and that, although I have validated much of the information with various health professionals in the field, I am basing a lot of it on my understanding and observations during my own recovery and in relation to my accounts of individuals who have suffered from similar conditions.

6.   Research News, 'Excessive growth of bacteria may also be major cause of stomach ulcers,' *Howard Hughes Medical Institute*, 15 January 2002, www.hhmi.org/news/merchant.html#top; Jim English, 'Heartburn and gastritis not always caused by too much acid: restoring gastric acid balance,' Worldwide Health Center, 17 November 2002, www.worldwidehealthcenter.net/ articles-225.html

7.   Ablation of the gallbladder is one of the most common surgical procedures in North America. Dr Lee suggests that gallbladder diseases are perhaps created by the hormonal imbalance resulting from oestrogen dominance; 20.5 million people are estimated to have had gallstones between 1988 and 1994 in the United States, according to the National Digestive Diseases Information Clearing House (NDDIC), http://digestive.niddk.nih.gov/statistics/statistics. htm#specific based on the study by J. E. Everhart, M. Khare, M. Hill and K. R. Maurer, 'Prevalence and ethnic differences in gallbladder disease in the United States,' *Gastroenterolog*, 1999, 117: 632–639; See also John Lee, J. Hanley and V. Hopkins, *What Your Doctor Won't Tell You About Premenopause*, New York, Warners Books, 1999, p.46.

8.   It could be another strain: *glabrata, krusei, parpsilopsis* or *tropicalis*.

9.   Alan R. Gaby, *The Natural Pharmacy: A Complete A–Z Reference to Natural Treatments for Common Health Conditions* (3rd edition), New York, Three Rivers Press, 2006, p.110.

10. Paul Pitchford, *Healing with Whole Foods*, Berkeley, CA, North Atlantic Books, 2002, p.73; Antibiotics alter the intestinal flora and cause the 'good bacteria' to disappear along with the undesirable bacteria. Prescriptions of probiotics issued by doctors have been growing in Quebec in response to the increasingly invasive problems of bacteria that is resistant to antibiotics in Quebec hospitals and the massive use of antibiotics. The results have been positive.

11. Paul Pitchford, *Healing with Whole Foods*, Berkeley, CA, North Atlantic Books, 2002, pp.71–73; Alan R. Gaby *The Natural Pharmacy: A Complete A–Z Reference to Natural Treatments for Common Health Conditions* (3rd edition), New York, Three Rivers Press, 2006, pp.109–111; James L. Wilson, *Adrenal Fatigue: The 21st Century Stress Syndrome*, Petaluma, CA, Smart Publications, 2001, chapters 5 and 6; 'Vitamin and mineral supplement fact sheet,' Office of Dietary Supplements, *National Institute of Health*, http://ods.od.nih.gov/Health_Information/Vitamin_and_Mineral_ Supplement_Fact_Sheets.aspx; Carolyn Dean, *The Miracle of Magnesium*, New York, Ballantine Books, 2003.

12. Gailon Totheoh, 'What's in that? How food affects behaviour,' *CBC News Science & Medical*, 1 July 2008. You can find the article and the video on www.cbn.com/CBNnews/353246.aspx.

13. Environment News Service, 'Pharmaceuticals found in drinking water,' www.monitor.net/monitor/9805a/drugwater.html (beta-blocker); Mike Adams, 2004, 'Antidepressant drugs found in drinking water; pharmaceuticals have now become environmental pollutants,' www.newstarget.com/001891.html (antidepressants); Janet Pelley, 'Nitrate eyed as endocrine disruptor,' Environmental Science & Technology, 2003, vol 37 (9), p.162A, and www.pubs.acs.org/action/doSearch?action=search&author=Pelley%2C+Janet; S. R. Hutchins, M. V. White, D. D. Fine and G. P. Breidenbach, 2003, Analysis of swine lagoons and ground water for environmental oestrogens, *Proceedings, Battelle In Situ and On-Site Bioremediation Symposium,* 2–5 June 2003, Orlando, FL (oestrogen); Janet Raloff, 'More "waters test positive for drugs",' *Science News Online,* 1 April 2000, vol 17, no 0212 (multi-residue); In London, in an effort to determine the population's cocaine consumption, scientists have detected an average of two kilograms of this drug emptied daily into the Thames. This is an economical way of getting a cheap fix. Information taken from the article, 5 August 2005, 'Where rivers run high on cocaine,' *The Times* and the article on cocaine that appeared in *ABC Newsonline* (2005) 'Cocaine traces detected in River Thames: report,' www.telegraph.co.uk/news/uknews/3325948/The-Thames-awash-with-cocaine.html. Studies carried out in 2008 by researchers at Université de Montréal on the water in the St Lawrence River show that the concentration of hormone disruptors was 90 to 100 times higher than the known rate. The reproductive organs in fish are greatly affected. What do our researchers say? Puberty is starting younger and younger in girls and clinics are popping up everywhere to deal with infertility in both men and women. Sexual hormones also play a major role in our mood and behaviour. Information drawn from 'Estrogen levels skyrocket in river around Montreal,' CBC, 17 September 2008, www.cbc.ca/health/story/2008/09/17/estrogen-stlawrence.html (hormone disruptors).

14. 'Maisonneuve en direct,' www.radio-canada.ca/radio/maisonneuve/19112004/42368.shtml.

15. The COX-1 enzyme possibly does it too, but in a very mild manner. For more information, see J. Fuchs and L. Packer, *Oxidative Stress and Disease,* Los Angeles, Marcel Dekker, 2001, p.244.

16. Paul Pitchford, *Healing with Whole Foods,* Berkeley, CA, North Atlantic Books, 2002, pp.171–173.

17. It is interesting to note that cortisol (stress hormone) is the main anti-inflammatory substance in the human body. If the adrenal glands are tired from battling a long inflammatory process (an auto-immune disease or something else), what will result will be an insufficient production of cortisol, which will then increase the inflammatory process, creating a vicious circle.

18. R. Béliveau and D. Gingras, *Les aliments contre le cancer,* Outremont, Éditions du Trécarré, 2005.

19. Zoltan P. Rona, 'Altered immunity & leaky gut syndrome,' www.afpafitness.com/articles/altered-immunity-leaky-gut-syndrome/85

20. T. Randolph and R. Moss, *An Alternative Approach to Allergies* (revised edition), New York, Harper and Row, 1990.

21. Here are some useful references: Association québécoise des allergies alimentaires, www.aqaa.qc.ca/index.htm; The world's healthiest foods, www.whfoods.com/genpage.php?tname=diet&dbid=7#research; Children's nutrition: J. Shulman, *Winning the Food Fight,* Etobicoke, John Wiley & Sons Canada Ltd, 2003; Janine Fontaine, *Les Maux méprisés,* Paris, Robert Laffont, 1992; T. Randolph, and R. Moss, *An Alternative Approach to Allergies* (revised edition), New York, Harper and Row, 2000; Canadian Food Inspection Agency, www.inspection.gc.ca

22. T. Randolph and R. Moss, *An Alternative Approach to Allergies* (revised edition), New York, Harper and Row, 2000; W. H. Philpott and D. K. Kalita, *Brain Allergies* (2nd edition), Chicago, Keats Publishing, 2000.

23. The Hypoglycemia Support Foundation, www.hypoglycemia.org/ or Association des hypoglycémiques du Québec, www.hypoglycemie.qc.ca

24. W. H. Philpott and D. K. Kalita, *Brain Allergies* (2nd edition), Chicago, Keats Publishing, 2000.

25. Pitchford, Paul, *Healing with Whole Foods,* Berkeley, CA, North Atlantic Books, 2002, p.245.

26. Xylitol and stevia leaves don't have this negative effect.

27. You will find a list of foods and their glycemic index at www.diabetesnet.com/diabetes_food_diet/glycemic_index.php#axzz13J3qMq00

28. W. H. Philpott and D. K. Kalita, *Brain Allergies* (2nd edition), Chicago, Keats Publishing, 2000, pp.148–149.

29. Philpott and Kalita, 2000, p.147.

30. Association des hypoglycémiques du Québec.

31. R. Béliveau and D. Gingras, *Les aliments contre le cancer*, Outremont, Éditions du Trécarré, 2005.

32. Studies on adrenal gland extracts taken orally have been mainly conducted in animals. The use of the bovine thymus extract has been scientifically studied. It is effective in preventing infection of the upper respiratory routes. For more information, see Alan R. Gaby, *The Natural Pharmacy: A Complete A–Z Reference to Natural Treatments for Common Health Conditions* (3rd edition), New York, Three Rivers Press, 2006.

33. For scientific information on homeopathy, see Bill Gray, *L'Homéopathie enfin prouvée!*, Paris, Guy Trédaniel Éditeur, 2002 and Glasgow Homoeopathic Hospital, 1053, Great Western Road, Glasgow G12 0XQ, Scotland, UK, Tel. 44 141 211 1617 Email hom-inform@dial.pipex.com

34. According to a laboratory test report dating back to 2003, 30 per cent of 20 probiotic products tested (12 refrigerated and 8 non-refrigerated) were contaminated, 50 per cent of non-refrigerated products wre completely dead. For more information, see D. Ingels and A. Gaby, 'Quality of probiotic supplements questioned: are you getting what you pay for?,' *A Healthnotes Newswire Opinion*, 2003, www.newhope.com/news.cfm?news=1257.

35. Paul Pitchford, *Healing with Whole Foods*, Berkeley, CA, North Atlantic Books, 2002, p.9.

36. Alan R. Gaby, *The Natural Pharmacy: A Complete A–Z Reference to Natural Treatments for Common Health Conditions* (3rd edition), New York, Three Rivers Press, 2006, pp.171–172.

37. M. Hornyak *et al.* 'Magnesium therapy for periodic leg movements-related insomnia and restless legs syndrome: An open pilot study,' *Sleep*, 1998, 21: 501–505; L. Popoviciu *et al.*, Clinical, EEG, electromyographic and polysomnographic studies in restless legs syndrome caused by magnesium deficiency,' *Rom J Neurol Psychiatry*, 1993, 31: 55–61.

38. Alan R. Gaby, 'Intravenous nutrient therapy: the "Myers" cocktail,' *Alternative Medicine Review*, 2002, 7(5): 389–403.

39. Carolyn Dean, *The Miracle of Magnesium*, New York, Ballantine Books, 2003, Chapter 9; Alan R. Gaby, *The Natural Pharmacy: A Complete A–Z Reference to Natural Treatments for Common Health Conditions* (3rd edition), New York, Three Rivers Press, 2006, p.113.

40. According to scientific documentation, tests of the magnesium concentration commonly used – in serum form or in blood plasma – are indicators that do not reflect the magnesium concentration in tissue, with the exception of interstitial fluid: this is therefore not valid data to effectively recognize a magnesium deficiency, given that 99 per cent of magnesium in the body is contained in the intracellular environment.

41. Alan R. Gaby, 'Magnesium deficiency associated with insulin-resistance syndrome,' *HealthNotes Newswire* 12 June 2003.

42. The magnesium website, www.mgwater.com

43. K.I. Peverill, L.A. Sparrow, D.J. Reuter, 'Soil analysis: an interpretation manual,' Collingwood, Csiro Publishing, 1999, p.255.

44. Carolyn Dean, *The Miracle of Magnesium*, New York, Ballantine Books, 2003.

45. Food and Agriculture Organisation of the United Nations: www.fao.org/DOCREP/004/Y2809E/y2809e0k.htm

46. For magnesium analysis alternatives, refer to www.exatest.com

47. The Canadian Office of Dietary Supplements website will give you an idea of the quantity of magnesium to take as a supplement, based on your age and your gender. This data is very conservative compared to the quantity that would be beneficial to a person who has been exhausted over a long period: http://ods.od.nih.gov/factsheets/Magnesium-HealthProfessional

48. Carolyn Dean, *The Miracle of Magnesium*, New York, Ballantine Books, 2003.

49. Use a good-quality inverted osmosis filter or a Doulton-type porcelain filter.

50. Avoid plastic containers. Choose glass or stainless-steel containers instead.

51. For the Greater Montreal Area, the *Pharmacie Pearson & Alter* specializes in these types of products: www.montrealpharmacy.com/english and www.fao.org/DOCREP/004/Y2809E/y2809e0k.htm

52. Candace Pert, *Molecules of Emotion*, New York, Touchstone, 1997, p.299.

Chapter 6

1. C. Chan, 'Neurophysiology course handout,' School of Physical and Occupational Therapy, McGill University, Canada, 1984–1985, p.3.
2. See World Research Foundation 'The electrical pattern of life; the work of Harold S. Burr,' www.wrf.org/men-women-medicine/dr-harold-s-burr.php; Rupert Sheldrake, biologist and author, www.sheldrake.org/homepage.html.
3. V. V. Hunt, *Infinite Mind* (2nd edition), Malibu, CA, Malibu Publishing, 1996, p.244; to learn more, see Jean-Marie Danze, 'La bioélectrographie GDV (Gaz Discharge Visualisation) by Professor Konstantin Korotkov,' 2007, www.plocher.fr and Konstantin Korokov on his website, www.korotkov.org
4. International Institute of Biophysics, German research groups, Neuss, Germany, http://www.lifescientists.de/ib0200e_.htm.
5. The emission of biophotons had initially been discovered by professor Alexander G. Gurvitch in 1923.
6. T. Amano, M. Kobayashi, B. Devaraj, M. Usa and H. Inaba, 'Ultraweak biophoton emission imaging of transplanted bladder cancer,' *Urological research*, vol. 23, no. 5, November 1995.
7. Lynn McTaggart, *The Field*, New York, Harper Perennial, pp.39–43.
8. J. Slawinski, M. Godlewski, T. Kwiecinska, Z. Rajfur, D. Sitko and D. Wierzuchowska, 'Stress-induced photon emission from perturbed organisms: Biophoton emission, stress and disease,' *Experientia*, 1992, vol. 48, no. 11–12: 1041–1058. T. Ohya, N. Oikawa, R. Kawabata, H. Okabe and S. Kai, 'Biophoton emission induced by osmotic stress in adzuki bean root,' Jpn J Appl Phys, Part 1, 2003, vol.42, no.12: 7625–7628.
9. Lynn McTaggart, *The Field*, New York, Harper Perennial, 2002, p.52.
10. W. Arntz, B. Chasse and M. Vicente, *Que sait-on vraiment de la réalité*, Outremont, Ariane, 2007.
11. Emotto Masuru, www.masaru-emoto.net
12. For more information, visit the website of the California Institute for Human Science, www.cihs.edu/whatsnew/research.asp.
13. Stephen Sagar, *Restored Harmony: An Evidence Based Approach for Integrating Traditional Chinese Medicine into Complementary Cancer Care*, Etobicoke, Dreaming Dragon Fly Communications, 2001.
14. Z. H. Cho, S. C. Chung, J. P. Jones *et al.* 'New findings of the correlation between acupoints and corresponding brain cortices using functional MRI,' *Proc Natl Acad Sci USA*, 1998, 95: 2670–2673.
    A. Alavi., P. J. LaRiccia., A. H. Sadek *et al.* 'Neuroimaging of acupuncture in patients with chronic pain,' *J Alt Comp Med*, 1997, 3 (suppl 1): S47–S53.
15. Paul B. Fitzgerald, Sarah Fountain and Zafiris J. Daskalakis, 'A comprehensive review of the effects of rTMS on motor cortical excitability and inhibition,' *Clinical Neurophysiology*, December 2006, 117(12): 2584–2596.
16. Or'ions, Bricard Law, www.info-systel.com/bricard_.en.html.
17. V. V. Hunt, *Infinite Mind* (2nd edition), Malibu, Malibu Publishing, 1996, p.26.
18. For more information, see C. Y. Shaw and G. T. Tamura, 'Air ions and human comfort,' *Canadian Building Digests, NRC-IRC Publications*, Canada, 1978, www.nrc-cnrc.gc.ca/eng/ibp/irc/cbd/building-digest-199.html.
19. Anu Karinen *et al.* 'Mobile phone radiation might alter protein expression in human skin,' *BMC Genomics*, February 11 2008, 9: 77.
20. To find out more about the effects of these waves, refer to www.powerwatch.org.uk; Duncan Graham-Rowe, 'Cancer cell study revives cell phone safety fears,' *New Scientist*, 2002, www.newscientist.com/article.ns?id=dn2959; article on the effects of an antenna used to pick up waves for cell phones on the dwellers of the tower where the antenna is situated, London Evening Standard, www.thisislondon.co.uk/news/article-23407354-details/Orange+to+remove+mobile+mast+from+%27tower+of+doom%27%2C+where+cancer+rate+has+soared/article.do.
21. J. Nadel and J. Decety, 'Résonance et agentivité,' *Cerveau & Psycho*, no. 13, February 2006.
22. Candace Pert, *Molecules of Emotion*, New York, Touchstone, 1997, p.312.
23. D. C. McClelland and C. Kirshnit, 'The effect of motivational arousal through films on salivary immunoglobulin A,' *Psychology and Health*, 2: 31–52.

24. K. M. Dillon *et al.* 'Positive emotional states and enhancement of the immune system,' *International Journal of Psychiatry in Medicine*, vol. 15 (1985–1988): 13–17.
G. Rein and R. McCraty, 'Long-term effects of compassion on salivary IgA,' *Psychosomatic Medicine*, vol. 56, 1994: 171–172.

25. Candace Pert, *Molecules of Emotion*, New York, Touchstone, 1997, p.23.

26. It is important for health professionals to note that there is a high concentration of these substances in the *brainstem* in which are located several nuclei linked to the senses that interact between themselves and with the nuclei that control the ANS rhythms. The areas of the body in which these concentrations are located have been called *nodal points.*

27. If you want to find out more about these energy and information theories, I suggest you read Lynn McTaggart, *The Field*, New York, Harper Perennial, 2002, and visit the website of Dr Stuart Hameroff, *The New Frontier in Brain/Mind Science*, www.quantumconsciousness.org/publications.html.

28. W. Arntz, B. Chasse and M. Vicente, *Que sait-on vraiment de la réalité?*, Outremont, Ariane, 2007.

29. Paul Pearsall, *The Heart's Code*, New York, Broadway Books, 1998.

30. B. Brewitt *et al.* 'The efficacy of reiki hands-on healing: improvements in spleen and nervous system function as quantified by electrodermal screening,' *Alternative Therapies*, July 1997, vol. 3, no. 4: 89.
Stephen Sagar, *Restored Harmony: An Evidence Based Approach for Integrating Traditional Chinese Medicine into Complementary Cancer Care*, Etobicoke, Dreaming Dragon Fly Communications, 2001.

31. Janice Bell Meisenhelder, 'Prayer and health outcomes in church lay leaders,' *Western Journal of Nursing Research*, 2002, vol. 22, no. 6: 706–716.

32. Lee Myeong Soo, Huh Hwa Jeong *et al.* 'Effects of emitted qi on in vitro natural killer,' *American Journal of Chinese Medicine*, 2001, 29: 17–22, http://findarticles.com/p/articles/mi_m0HKP/is_1_29/ai_73711239/?tag=content;col1; The Intention Experiment, www.theintentionexperiment.com/the_experiments.

Chapter 7

1. Robert Musil, *The Confusions of Young Törless*, Pantheon Books, 1906.

2. To learn more about the theories of how ANS works and the vagus nerve component related to the brain stem: see S. W. Porges, 'Orienting in a defensive world: mammalian modification of our evolutionary heritage, a polyvagal theory,' *Psychophysiology*, 32 (1995): 301–318.

3. I often encounter this problem in my clients suffering from degenerative neurological diseases. Once the neurovegetative rhythms are better controlled in therapy, what results is a sense of well-being and increased energy despite the disease.

4. M. A. Haxhiu *et al.* 'The brainstem network in coordination of inspiratory activity and cholinergic outflow to the airways,' *J Auton Nerv Syst*, 1996, 61(2): 155–161.

5. It is normal to have a residual volume of air in the lungs, even after a deep breath, but this volume is minimal compared to that found in chest breathing.

6. Charles Krebs, *A Revolutionary way of Thinking*, Melbourne, Hill of Content, 1998, chapter 6 and p.224.

7. S. A. Jella and D. S. Shannahoff-Khalsa, 'The effects of unilateral forced nostril breathing on cognitive performance,' *Int J Neurosci*, 1993, 73(1–2): 61–68; B. B. Schiff and S. A. Rump, 'Asymmetrical hemispheric activation and emotion: the effects of unilateral forced nostril breathing,' *Brain Cogn*, 1995, 29(3): 217–231.

8. Course notes from *Formation à la méthode Padovan de réorganisation neurofonctionnelle: Module II – Les fonctions orofaciales et leur rééducation* by Beatriz Padovan and Sônia Padovan-Catenne, November 2005.

9. For more details on breathing control, see Arthur Guyton, *Anatomie et physiologie du système nerveux*, Montréal, Décary Éditeur, 1989, p.376.

10. If you are interested in learning more about the heart from an energy perspective, refer to the book by Paul Pearsall, *The Heart's Code*, New York, Broadway Books, 1998.

11. J. Shulman, *Winning the Food Fight*, Etobicoke, John Wiley & Sons Canada Ltd, 2003.

12. Many people suffering from energy disorders can experience a very tight jaw and neck. Scientific documentation now shows that many people afflicted with fibromyalgia suffer from temporomandibular joint dysfunction, since this joint is associated with our postural adjustments and suction, chewing and swallowing rhythms.

13. Michael Hasting, 'The brain, circadian rhythms, and clock genes,' *British Medical Journal*, 317, 1998: 19–26.

14. Article by Daniel Baril on the work of Mario Beauregard in functional magnetic resonance on the brains of Carmelites, 'Il n'existe pas de module de Dieu dans le cerveau,' *Université de Montréal, Forum*, vol. 41, no. 1, 28 August 2006, www.iforum.umontreal.ca/Forum/2006-2007/20060828/R_3.html; Ulrich Kraft, 'La neurobiologie de la méditation,' *Cerveau & Psycho: Le magazine de la psychologie et des neurosciences*, 13, 2006: 4650.

15. You only have to read the article by Marie Lambert-Chan in *La Presse*, July 28, 2007, on 'Les vertus de la sieste au travail'. The article reports that the consulting firm Deloitte & Touche had to close its room reserved for naps. Although the experiment revealed itself to be conclusive as to the level of productivity, it gave the firm too much negative press for it to be able to continue with this practice.

16. P. Lalonde, F. Grunberg *et al. Psychiatrie clinique: approche bio-psycho-sociale*, Montréal: Gaëtan Morin Éditeur, 1988, p.408. This hormone is also called Adrenocorticotrophic Hormone (ACTH).

17. James L. Wilson, *Adrenal Fatigue: The 21st Century Stress Syndrome*, Petaluma, CA, Smart Publications, 2001, p.266.

18. Hans Selye, *The Stress of Life*, New York: McGraw-Hill Paperbacks, 1956, p.177.

19. Hans Selye, Ibid, p.178.

20. L. Lee, J. Hanley and V. Hopkins *What Your Doctor Won't Tell You About Premenopause*, New York, Warners Books, 1999, p.177.

21. B. Malpaux, C. Viguié, J. C. Thiéry and P. Chemineau, 'Contrôle photopériodique de la reproduction,' *INRA Productions animales*, 1996, 9: 9–23.

22. For very severe cases of sympathic/parasympathic imbalance, the neurofunctional reorganization method performed with a qualified professional yields quick results from the initial sessions.

23. It is possibly not a coincidence that smokers, given that they are stimulated by nicotine, find the act of inhaling and exhaling cigarette smoke subjectively relaxing. In addition to the breathing phenomenon, smoking indirectly mimics the sucking reflex.

24. A. O. Massion *et al.* 'Meditation, melatonin and breast/prostate cancer: hypothesis and preliminary data,' *Medical Hypotheses*, 44, 1995, 39–46; G. A. Tooley *et al.* 'Acute increases in night-time plasma melatonin levels following a period of meditation,' *Biological Psychology*, 53, 2000, 69–78; E. Leskowitz, 'Seasonal affective disorder and the yoga paradigm: a reconsideration of the role of the pineal gland,' *Medical Hypotheses*, 33, 1990, 155–158.

25. Refer to www.ergoenergie.com.

26. The method is very well explained in the book by Shou-Yu Liang and Wu Wen-Ching, *Simplified Tai Chi Chuan with Applications: 24 & 48 Postures with Martial Applications*. Washington, YMAA Publication Center, 1996.

27. N. Alexandros *et al.* 'Chronic insomnia is associated with nyctrohemeral activation of the hypothalamic-pituitary-adrenal axis: clinical implications,' *Journal of Clinical Endocrinology and Metabolism*, 2001, 86: 3787–3794.

28. David Servan-Schreiber, *Healing Without Freud or Prozac: Natural Approaches to Curing Stress, Anxiety and Depression without Drugs and without Psychoanalysis*, Emmaus, PA, Rodale Press, 2005, chapter 4.

29. Marie Dumont, 'Strategies for shiftworkers,' *Canadian Sleep Society*, 2003.

30. J. Lee, J. Hanley and V. Hopkins, *What Your Doctor May Not Tell You About Premenopause*, New York, Warner Books, 1999 and www.johnleemd.com

Chapter 8

1. Gary Kielhofner, *A Model of Human Occupation*, Baltimore, Williams & Wilkins, 1985, and course notes of Gary Kielhofner, *The model of human occupation applied to psychiatry*, Ottawa Civic Hospital, 1987.
2. Eckhart Tolle, *Le pouvoir du moment présent*, Outremont, Ariane Éditions, 2000, chapter 3.
3. Eckhart Tolle, *Le pouvoir du moment présent*, Outremont, Ariane Éditions, 2000.
4. Information is a form of energy, as explained in Chapter 6.
5. Eckhart Tolle, *Le pouvoir du moment présent*, Outremont, Ariane Éditions, 2000, chapter 3; Krishnamurti spoke more or less of the same thing when he was explaining the external time (clock or chronological) and inner time (psychological): Krishnamurti, *La flamme de l'attention*, London, Éditions du Rocher, 1987, p.50.
6. On a neurological level, this activity is, for many of my patients, one of the best ways of restoring the sympathetic/parasympathetic balance, because it triggers a great number of ANS rhythms (breathing, suction, chewing, swallowing, and peristalsis). In addition, it contains a rich source of info-energy for the senses. I was very pleased to see that the therapists who use the mindfulness meditation method, a method that has been proven in the context of stress management, also suggest this type of exercise. For more information, visit the website of the School of Medicine of the University of Massachusetts, www.umassmed.edu/behavmed/faculty/kabat-zinn.cfm.
7. Elisabeth Kübler-Ross, *The Real Taste of Life: A Photographic Journal*, 1969.
8. Eckhart Tolle, *The Power of Now*, Vancouver, Namaste Publishing Library, 2004, p.96.

Chapter 9

1. Gorun Arnadòttir, *The Brain and Behavior*, St Louis, C. V. Mosby Company, 1990, p.314.
2. Winnie Dunn, 'The sensations of everyday life: empirical, theoretical and pragmatic considerations,' *American Journal of Occupational Therapy*, November/December 2001, vol. 55, no. 6, pp.608–620.
3. Winnie Dunn, Ibid, pp.608–620.
4. The example that I see most frequently in my practice is that of temporomandibular joint dysfunction (TMJD) in exhausted people, and the repercussions on posture and the autonomous nervous system.
5. Quoted by Michael Jawer, 'Environmental sensitivity: a neurobiological phenomenon?' Seminar in Integrative Medicine, *Point of View: Elsevier*, 2005, pp.104–109.
6. For more details, refer to Charles Krebs, *A Revolutionary Way of Thinking*, Melbourne, Hill of Content, 1998.
7. Charles Krebs, 1998, chapter 4.
8. It is certain that when one suffers from incapacitating persistent fatigue, intense physical exercise is not recommended. To estimate the level of physical effort that can be tolerated without exacerbating the condition, consult Chapter 4.
9. A. Lutz, L. Greischar, N. Rawling, M. Ricard and R. Davidson, 'Long-term meditators self-induce high-amplitude gamma synchrony during mental practice,' *Proceedings of the National Academy of Sciences of the United States of America*, 2004, 101: 16369–16373 and P. Reuter-Lorenz and Richard J. Davidson, 'Deferential contributions of the two cerebral hemispheres to the perception of happy and sad faces,' *Neurophychologia*, vol. 19, no. 4, 1981: 609–613.
10. Through techniques focused on consciousness of the self such as those suggested in Chapters 8 and 12, it is possible to increase the ratio of left cerebral activation compared to the right side and favourably affect the emotional response. See R. J. Davidson *et al.* 'Alterations in brain and immune function produced by mindfulness meditation,' *Psychomatic Medicine*, 65, 2003: 564–570.
11. *Modern Synopsis of Comprehensive Textbook of Psychiatry/III* (3rd edition), Baltimore, Williams & Wilkins, 1981, pp.132–136.
12. M. Seligman, *Learned Optimism: How to Change Your Mind and Your Life*, New York, Vintage, 2006, p.282.

13. To explore this topic in greater depth, see David R. Hawkins, *The Eye Of The I: From Which Nothing is Hidden*, Sedona, Veritas Publishing, 2001.
14. We will return to this issue in greater detail in Chapter 11 to find the motivations underlying our thoughts.
15. I am summarizing here the observations of Dr Seligman and his colleagues, which are used extensively in cognitive behavioral therapy. For further details, see M. Seligman, *Learned Optimism: How to Change Your Mind and Your Life*, New York, Vintage, 2006.
16. To deepen optimism, refer to M. Seligman, ibid.
17. David Burns, *Feeling Good: The New Mood Therapy* (revised and updated), New York, Avon Books, 1999.

Chapter 10

1. Some people need a psychologist to carry out this basic cleansing. For those without the financial means, I strongly suggest the book by David Burns, *Feeling Good: The New Mood Therapy* (revised and updated), New York, Avon Books, 1999.
2. Mary Ann McColl, *Spirituality and Occupational Therapy*, Ottawa, CAOT, 2003, p.91.

Chapter 11

1. I have chosen the word *power* because in physics the concept of *power* refers to the concept of energy.
2. Translated from Serge Mongeau, *La Simplicité volontaire, plus que jamais…*, Montréal, Les Éditions Écosociété, 1998, p.170.
3. Translated from Etty Buzyn, *Papa, maman, laissez-moi le temps de rêver*, Paris, Albin Michel, 1995, p.74.
4. Canadian data from the years 1994–1995 to 2000–2001 based on the analysis exposed by sociologist Alain Marchand at the convention of AIISTQ on work conditions and personalities, 30 April 2008.
5. Katherine Marchall, 'Study: on sick leave,' *The Daily*, 21 April 2006, www.statcan.gc.ca/daily-quotidien/060421/dq060421d-eng.htm; Nicolas Chevrier and Sonia Renon-Chevrier, 'L'épuisement professionnel: Vers des interventions organisationnels.' *Psychologie Québec*, November 2004: 39–40.
6. Fletcher quoted in J. A. Davis, 'An occupation perspective on work-life balance,' *Occupational Therapy Now*, 6(3), 2004: 20–21.
7. Ibid.
8. Ibid.
9. Bernie S. Siegel, *Love, Medicine and Miracles*, New York, Harper & Row, 1986, p.87.
10. Mary Ann McColl, *Spirituality and Occupational Therapy*, Ottawa, CAOT, 2003, chapter 2.
11. David R. Hawkins, *I: Reality And Subjectivity*, West Sedona, Veritas Publishing, 2003, p.72.
12. E. Townsend, S Banks, L. Multari and A. Naugh, *OT Guidelines for Client-Centred Practice*, Toronto, CAOT, 1991, p.58.

Chapter 12

1. McGill University on the triune brain: 'The brain from top to bottom,' http://thebrain.mcgill.ca; J. Kiernan, *Barr's The Human Nervous System: An Anatomical Viewpoint* (8th edition), Baltimore, Lippincott Williams & Wilkins, 2005; Charles Krebs, *A Revolutionary Way of Thinking*, Melbourne, Hill of Content, 1998; John Ratey, *A User's Guide to the Brain*, New York, First Vintage Books, 1994.
2. Also called *primitive*.

3. For therapists and interested parties, being very familiar with the way in which the brainstem works is an asset. You will be able to monitor the surprising changes that awareness of the body and of its rhythms induces to bring about a return to *homeostasis* of all the interconnected systems. In my practice, it is the best access door for regulating the ANS functions and reestablishes its rhythms. A notable impact will result, among other things there will be a major impact on the hypothalamic-pituitary-adrenal axis.

4. P. J. Whorwell *et al.* 'Physiological effects of emotion: assessment via hypnosis,' *Lancet*, 1992, 340(8811): 69–72; W. M. Gonsalkorale, V. Miller, A. Afzal and P. J. Whorwell, 'Long term benefits of hypnotherapy for irritable bowel syndrome,' *Gut*, 2003, 52: 1623–1629; B. Goldberg, 'Hypnosis and the immune response,' *Int. J. Psychosom*, 1985, 32(3): 34–36; effectiveness of hypnosis and relaxation in children suffering from migraines, www. adrenaline112.org/hypnose/doul/doulmigrenf.html.

5. Canadian Psychological Association, www.cpa.ca/home and American Psychological Association, on www.apa.org

6. Shakti Gawain, *Creative Visualization*, Novato, New World Library, 2002.

7. F. Stetter and S. Kupper, 'Autogenic training: a meta-analysis of clinical outcome studies,' *Appl Psychophysiol Biofeedback*, 2002, 27(1): 45–98; N. Kanji, 'Management of pain through autogenic training,' *Complement Ther Nurs Midwifery*, 2000, 6(3): 143–148.

8. Canadian Association of Acupuncture & Traditional Chinese Medicine, www.caatcm. com/?page_id=171

9. David Servan-Schreiber, *Guérir: le stress, l'anxiété et la dépression sans médicaments ni psychanalyse*, Paris, Robert Laffont, 2003, chapter 4; Paul Pearsall, *The Heart's Code*, New York, Broadway Books, 1998.

10. T. Field, M. Hernandez-Reif, M. Diego, S. Schanberg and C. Kunh, 'Cortisol decreases and serotonin and dopamine increase following massage therapy,' *Int J Neurosci*, 2005, 115(10): 1397–1413.

11. To learn more about the benefits of touching, I recommend A. Montagu, *Touching: The Human Significance of the Skin* (2nd edition), New York, Harper & Row Publishers, 1978.

12. David Servan-Schreiber, *Guérir: le stress, l'anxiété et la dépression sans médicaments ni psychanalyse*, Paris, Robert Laffont, 2003, chapter 6.

13. Marc Kaufman, 'Meditation gives brain a charge, study finds,' *Washington Post*, 3 January 2005, p.A05, www.washingtonpost.com/wp-dyn/articles/A43006-2005Jan2.html; Ulrich Kraft, 'La neurobiologie de la méditation,' *Cerveau & Psycho*, 13, 2006, 946–949.

14. J. Kabat-Zinn, A Massion, J. Kristeller, L.G. Peterson, L. Fletcher, L. Pbert, W. Linderking and S. F. Santorelli, 'Effectiveness of a meditation-based stress reduction program in the treatment of anxiety disorders,' *An J Psychiatry*, 1992, 149: 936–943.

15. The International Feldenkrais Federation (IFF), www.feldenkrais-method.org

16. Feldenkrais Guild of North America, www.feldenkrais.com, the Feldenkrais Guild in UK, www. feldenkrais.co.uk, and Association Feldenkrais Québec, www.feldenkraisqc.info

17. C. Hopper *et al.* 'The effects of Feldenkrais awareness through movement on hamstring length, flexibility, and perceived exertion,' *Journal of Body and Movement Therapies*, 1999, 3(4): 238–247.

18. A good reference book on stretching is Bob Anderson, *Stretching* (revised edition), Bolinas, Shelter Publications, 2000.

19. In the case of myalgic encephalomyelitis, fibromyalgia, joint hypermobility or a long history of anxiety disorder, yoga is not recommended without the supervision of an occupational therapist or a physiotherapist. Yoga classes are often too demanding for people suffering from these medical conditions.

20. Padovan's method: www.padovan.pro.br/default_en.htm; Association québécoise de la méthode Padovan, www.padovan.ca/files; for Europe, www.padovan-synchronicite.fr/html/accueil.html.

21. H. M. Taggart *et al.* 'Effects of tai chi exercise on fibromyalgia symptoms and health-related quality of life,' *Orthop Nurs*, 2003, 22(5): 252–260.

22. For therapists, I want to indicate that many of these movements resemble proprioceptive neuromuscular facilitation exercises.

23. D. Xu, Y. Hong, J. Li and K. Chan, 'Effect of taichi exercises on proprioception of ankle and knee joints in old people,' *Department of Sport, Science and Physical Education, and Department of Orthopedics and Traumatology, The Chinese University of Hong Kong,* February 2003; P. M. Wayne *et al.* 'Can tai chi improve vestibulopathic postural control?,' *Arch Phy Med Rehab,* 85, 2004.

24. For more information on the PCPSP© program 2005 on managing stress, pain and persistent fatigue see www.ergoenergie.com.

25. P. Guitard, F. Ferland and É. Dutil, 'L'importance de l'attitude ludique en ergothérapie avec une clientèle adulte,' *CJOT,* 2006, 73(5).

Chapter 13

1. John Wass and Stephen Shalet, *Oxford Textbook of Endocrinology And Diabetes,* Bath, Oxford University Press, 2002, p.280; Hans Selye, *The Stress of Life,* New York, McGraw-Hill Paperbacks, 1956; John Lee, J. Hanley and V. Hopkins, *What your Doctor Won't Tell You About Premenopause,* New York, Warners Books, 1999; Stuart Fox, *Human Physiology,* Chicago, WCB, 1996, chapter 11.

2. Fox, Ibid, p.289.

3. J. Lee, J. Hanley and V. Hopkins, *What your Doctor Won't Tell You About Premenopause,* New York, Warners Books, 1999, chapter 5.

4. Ibid, p.82.

5. Ibid, p.141.

6. R. A. Bowen, L. Austgen and M. Rouge, 'Pathophysiology of the Endocrine System,' Department of Biomedical Sciences, Colorado State University, updated 30 April 2006 http://arbl.cvmbs.colostate.edu/hbooks/pathphys/endocrine/adrenal/steroids.html; Stuart Fox, *Human Physiology,* Chicago, WCB, 1996, chapter 11.

7. Yvan Labelle, *L'hypoglycémie: un dossier choc,* Montreal, Les Éditions fleurs sociales, 1989, chapter 6.

8. Glycogenolysis is the process in which glucose is released in its stored form of glycogen. Glycogenesis is the synthesis of glycogen using glucose for storage purposes. Only the cells of the liver and the muscle tissue can create these two processes.

9. Yvan Labelle, *L'hypoglycémie: un dossier choc,* Montreal, Les Éditions fleurs sociales, 1989, p.113.

10. John Lee, J. Hanley and V. Hopkins, *What Your Doctor Won't Tell You About Premenopause,* New York, Warners Books, 1999, p.46.

11. Dave Tuttle, 'Keeping a dangerous hormone in check,' *Life Extension,* July 2004.

12. Ridha Arem, *The Thyroid Solution,* Toronto, Random House Publishing, 1999, p.167.

13. Ibid, p.29.

14. www.townsendletter.com; www.adrenalfatigue.org

15. Candace Pert, Arem Ridha, Paul Pearsall, John Lee, and James L. Wilson.

References

Adams, D, *So Long, and Thanks for All the Fish*, London, Pan Macmillan, 1984.

Adams, Mike, 'Antidepressant drugs found in drinking water; pharmaceuticals have now become environmental pollutants,' *Natural News.com*, 2004, www.newstarget.com/001891.html, accessed December 2011.

Ainsworth, BE *et al.* 'Compendium of physical activities: classification of energy cost of human physical activities,' *Medicine and Science in Sports and Activities*, 1993; 25: 71–80.

Alavi, A, LaRiccia, PJ, Sadek, AH *et al.* 'Neuroimaging of acupuncture in patients with chronic pain,' *J Alt Comp Med*, 1997; 3 (suppl. 1): S47–S53.

Alexandros, N *et al.* 'Chronic insomnia is associated with nyctrohemeral activation of the hypothalamic-pituitary-adrenal axis: clinical implications,' *Journal of Clinical Endocrinology and Metabolism*, August 2001; 86: 3787–3794.

Amano, T, Kobayashi, M, Devaraj, B, Usa, M and Inaba, H, 'Ultraweak biophoton emission imaging of transplanted bladder cancer,' *Urological Research*, 1995; 23(5).

American Psychiatric Association, *Diagnostic and Statistical Manual of Mental Disorders* (4th edition), Washington, APA, 1994.

Anderson, Bob, *Stretching* (revised edition), Bolinas, Shelter Publications, 2000.

Arnadòttir, Gorun, *The Brain and Behavior*, St Louis, C. V. Mosby Company, 1990.

Arntz, W, Chasse, B, and Vicente, M, *Que sait-on vraiment de la réalité*, Outremont, Ariane, 2007.

Ayres, Jean, *Sensory Integration and Learning Disorders*, Los Angeles, CA, Western Psychological Services, 1972.

Baril, Daniel, 'Il n'existe pas de module de Dieu dans le cerveau,' *Université de Montréal, Forum*, 28 August 2006; 41(1), www.iforum.umontreal.ca/Forum/2006-2007/20060828/R_3.html, accessed December 2011.

Béliveau, R. and Gingras, D, *Les aliments contre le cancer*, Outremont, Éditions du Trécarré, 2005.

Bell Meisenhelder, J 'Prayer and health outcomes in church lay leaders,' *Western Journal of Nursing Research*, 2002; 22(6): 706–716.

Botham, Catherine, Homes, Philip and Harrison, Paul, 'Endocrine disruption in mammals, birds, reptiles and amphibians,' *Environmental Science and Technology*, 1999; 12.

Bowen, RA, Austgen, L and Rouge M, 'Pathophysiology of the endocrine system,' Department of Biomedical Sciences, Colorado State University, updated April 30, 2006, http://arbl.cvmbs.colostate.edu/hbooks/pathphys/endocrine/adrenal/steroids.html, accessed December 2011.

Brewitt, B *et al.* 'The efficacy of reiki hands-on healing: improvements in spleen and nervous system function as quantified by electrodermal screening,' *Alternative Therapies*, July 1997: 3(4): 89.

Burns, David, *Feeling Good: The New Mood Therapy* (revised and updated), New York, Avon Books, 1999.

Buzyn, Etty, Papa, maman, laissez-moi le temps de rêver, Paris, Albin Michel, 1995.

Casey, Susan, 'Plastic ocean,' *Best Life*, Feb 20, 2007, www.bestlifeonline.com/cms/publish/travel-leisure/Our_oceans_are_turning_into_plastic_are_we.shtml.

CBC, 'Estrogen levels skyrocket in river around Montreal,' September 17, 2008, www.cbc.ca/health/story/2008/09/17/estrogen-stlawrence.html, accessed December 2011.

Centers for Disease Control and Prevention, 'Measuring physical activity intensity,' www.cdc.gov/nccdphp/dnpa/physical/measuring/met.htm, accessed December 2011.

Chair in Occupational Health and Safety Management, Université Laval, 'Employee recognition,' 2006; www.cgsst.com/eng/whats-new-.asp, accessed December 2011.

Chan, C, 'Neurophysiology course handout,' School of Physical and Occupational Therapy, McGill University, 1984–5, p.3.

Chevrier, Nicolas, and Renon-Chevrier, Sonia, 'L'épuisement professionnel: vers des interventions organisationnels,' *Psychologie Québec*, Nov. 2004: 39–40.

Christensen, Larry B, *The Food-Mood Connection*, Texas, Pro-health Publications, 1991.

Danze, Jean-Marie, 'La Bioélectrographie GCV (Gaz Discharge Visualiùaation) by Professeur Konstantin Korotkov,' 2007; www.plocher.fr/, accessed December 2011.

Davidson, RJ *et al.* 'Alterations in brain and immune function produced by mindfulness meditation,' *Psychomatic Medicine*, 2003; 65: 564–570.

Davis, JA, 'An occupation perspective on work-life balance,' *Occupational Therapy Now*, 2004; 6(3): 20–21.

Dean, Carolyn, *The Miracle of Magnesium*, New York, Ballantine Books, 2003.

Desjardins Arnaud, *L'Audace de vivre*, Paris, La table ronde, 1989.

Dillon, KM *et al.* 'Positive emotional states and enhancement of the immune system,' *International Journal of Psychiatry in Medicine*, 15, 1985–6: 13–17.

Doc Monde Épisode, 'Le paradoxe démographique,' documentary, *Télé-Québec*, 16 April 2007.

Dumont, Marie, 'Strategies for shiftworkers,' *Canadian Sleep Society*, 2003.

Dunn Winnie, 'The sensations of everyday life: empirical, theoretical and pragmatic considerations,' *American Journal of Occupational Therapy*, November/December 2001; 55(6): 608–620.

Dyer, Wayne, Your Erroneous Zones, New York, Avon Books, 1976.

English, Jim, 'Heartburn and gastritis not always caused by too much acid: restoring gastric acid balance,' *Worldwide Health Center*, 2002; Nov. 17, www.worldwidehealthcenter.net/articles-225.html, accessed December 2011.

Environment News Service, 'Pharmaceuticals found in drinking water,' www.monitor.net/monitor/9805a/drugwater.html, accessed December 2011.

Everhart, E, Khare, M, Hill, M and Maurer, KR, 'Prevalence and ethnic differences in gallbladder disease in the United States,' *Gastroenterology*, 1999; 117:632–639.

Field, T, Hernandez-Reif, M, Diego, M, Schanberg, S and Kunh, C, 'Cortisol decreases and serotonin and dopamine increase following massage therapy,' *Int J Neurosci*, 2005; 115(10): 1397–1413.

Fitzgerald, P B, Fountain, S and Daskalakis, Z J, 'A comprehensive review of the effects of rTMS on motor cortical excitability and inhibition,' *Clinical Neurophysiology*, December 2006; 117(12): 2584–2596.

Fontaine, Janine, *Les Maux méprisés*, Paris, Robert Laffont, 1992.

Fontaine, Janine, *Nos trois corps et les trois mondes*, Paris, Robert Laffont, 1986.

Food and Agriculture Organisation of the United Nations: www.fao.org/DOCREP/004/Y2809E/y2809e0k.htm.

Fox, Stuart, *Human Physiology*, Chicago, WCB, 1996.

Fuchs, J and Packer, L, *Oxidative Stress and Disease*, Los Angeles, Marcel Dekker, 2001.

Gaby, Alan R, *The Natural Pharmacy: A Complete A–Z Reference to Natural Treatments for Common Health Conditions* (3rd edition), New York, Three Rivers Press, 2006.

Gaby, Alan R, 'Magnesium deficiency associated with insulin-resistance syndrome,' *Health Notes Newswire*, June 12, 2003.

Gaby, Alan R, 'Intravenous nutrient therapy: the 'Myers' cocktail,'' *Alternative Medicine Review*, 2002; 7(5): 389–403.

Gawain, Shakti, *Creative Visualization*, Novato, CA, New World Library, 2002.

Gonsalkorale, WM, Miller, V, Afzal, A, Whorwell, PJ, 'Long term benefits of hypnotherapy for irritable bowel syndrome,' *Gut*, Nov. 2003; 52: 1623–1629.

Gottschalk, LA, Rebello, T, Buchsbaum, MS, Ticker, HG and Hodges, EL, 'Abnormalities in hair trace elements as indicators of aberrant behavior,' *Compr Psychiatry*, 1991; 32(2): 229–237.

Graham-Rowe, Duncan, 'Cancer cell study revives cell phone safety fears,' *New Scientist*, 2002.

Gray, Bill, *L'Homéopathie enfin prouvée!*, Paris, Guy Trédaniel Éditeur, 2002.

Guitard, P, Ferland, F and Dutil É, 'L'importance de l'attitude ludique en ergothérapie avec une clientèle adulte,' CJOT, 2006; 73(5).

Guyton, Arthur C, *Anatomie et physiologie du système nerveux*, Montreal, Décary Éditeur, 1989.

Hasting, Michael, 'The brain, circadian rhythms, and clock genes,' *British Medical Journal*, Dec 1998; 317: 19–26.

Hawkins, David R, *I: Reality and Subjectivity*, West Sedona, Veritas Publishing, 2003.

Hawkins, David R, *Power versus Force: The Hidden Determinants of Human Behavior*, Carlsbad, Hay House, 2002.

Hawkins, David R. *The Eye of the I: From which Nothing is Hidden*, Sedona, Veritas Publishing, 2001.

Haxhiu, MA *et al*. 'The brainstem network in coordination of inspiratory activity and cholinergic outflow to the airways,' *J Auton Nerv Syst*, 1996; 61(2): 155–161.

Health Canada, 'Medically unexplained physical symptoms, *The Daily*, Friday, January 12th 2007, www.statcan.gc.ca/daily-quotidien/070112/dq070112b-eng.htm, accessed December 2011.

Holmes, TH and Rahe, RH, 'The social readjustment rating scale,' *Journal of Psychosomatic Research*, 1967; 11: 213–218.

Hopper, C *et al*. 'The effects of Feldenkrais awareness through movement on hamstring length, flexibility, and perceived exertion,' *Journal of Body and Movement Therapies*, 1999; 3(4): 238–247.

Hornyak, M *et al*. 'Magnesium therapy for periodic leg movements-related insomnia and restless legs syndrome: an open pilot study,' *Sleep*, 1998; 21: 501–505.

Horowitz, M *et al*. 'Life event questionnaires for measuring presumptive stress,' *Psychosomatic Medicine*, 1977; 39(6).

Howard Hughes Medical Institute, 'Excessive growth of bacteria may also be major cause of stomach ulcers,' *Research News*, January 15, 2002, www.hhmi.org/news/merchant.html#top, accessed December 2011.

Hunt, VV, *Infinite Mind: The Science of Human Vibrations of Consciousness* (2nd edition), Malibu, Malibu Publishing, 1996.

Hutchins, SR, White, MV, Fine, DD and Breidenbach, GP, 'Analysis of swine lagoons and ground water for environmental œstrogens,' *Proceedings, Battelle In Situ and On-Site Bioremediation Symposium,* June 2–5, 2003, Orlando, FL.

Ingels, D and Gaby, A, 'Quality of probiotic supplements questioned: are you getting what you pay for?,' *A Healthnotes Newswire Opinion*, 2003; www.newhope.com/news.cfm?news=1257, accessed December 2011.

Jacobson, EC, *Savoir relaxer*, Montreal: Les Éditions de l'homme, 1980.

Jaffe, Russel 'Food & chemical effects on acid/alkaline body chemical balance,' *Health Studies Collegium*, 2002.

Jawer, Michael, 'Environmental sensitivity: a neurobiological phenomenon?,' Seminar in Integrative Medicine, *Point of View: Elsevier*, 2005.

Jella, SA and Shannahoff-Khalsa, DS, 'The effects of unilateral forced nostril breathing on cognitive performance,' *Int J Neurosci*, 1993; 73(1–2): 61–68.

Jung, Carl, *Collected Works of C. G. Jung*, vol. 9, part 1, 2nd edition, Princeton, NJ, Princeton University Press, 1968.

Kabat-Zinn, J, Massion, A, Kristeller, J, Peterson, LG, Fletcher L, Pbert, L, Linderking, W and Santorelli, SF, 'Effectiveness of a meditation-based stress reduction program in the treatment of anxiety disorders,' *An J Psychiatry*, 1992; 149: 936–943

Kanji, N, 'Management of pain through autogenic training,' *Complement Ther Nurs Midwifery*, 2000; 6(3): 143–148.

Kaufman, Marc, 'Meditation gives brain a charge, study finds,' *Washington Post*, January 3, 2005; A05, www.washingtonpost.com/wp-dyn/articles/A43006-2005Jan2.html, accessed December 2011.

Karinen, Anu *et al.* 'Mobile phone radiation might alter protein expression in human skin,' *BMC Genomics*, Feb. 11, 2008; 9: 77.

Kielhofner, Gary, *A Model of Human Occupation*, Baltimore, Williams & Wilkins, 1985.

Kiernan, J, *Barr's The Human Nervous System: An Anatomical Viewpoint* (8th edition), Baltimore, Lippincott Williams & Wilkins, 2005.

King, Michael W 'The medical biochemistry page,' National Science Teachers Association, http://themedicalbiochemistrypage.org/, accessed December 2011.

Kraft, Ulrich, 'La neurobiologie de la méditation,' *Cerveau & Psycho*, 2006, 13: 946–949.

Kraus, K (1874–1936), Trans. by Harry Zohn, *Half-Truths and One-and-a-Half Truths*, Chicago, University of Chicago Press, 1990 (originally published in Beim Wort genommen, 1955).

Krebs, Charles, *A Revolutionary Way of Thinking*, Melbourne, Hill of Content, 1998.

Krishnamurti, *La flamme de l'attention*, London: Éditions du Rocher, 1987.

Kübler-Ross, E, *The Real Taste of Life: A Photographic Journal*, 1969.

Labelle, Yvan, *L'hypoglycémie: un dossier choc!*, Montreal, Les Éditions fleurs sociales, 1989.

Lalonde, P, Grunberg, F. *et al. Psychiatrie clinique: approche bio-psycho-sociale,* Montreal, Gaëtan Morin Editeur, 1988.

Lambert-Chan, Marie, 'Les vertus de la sieste au travail,' *La Presse*, Saturday, July 28, 2007.

Languirand, Jacques, *Vaincre le burnout*, Montreal, Stanké, 2002.

Law, M, Baptiste, S, Carswell, A, McColl, MA, Polatajko, H and Pollock, N, *The Canadian Occupational Performance Measure*, Ottawa, Publications ACE, 1994.

Lee, J, Hanley, J and Hopkins, V, *Tout savoir sur la préménopause,* Vannes, Sully, 2001.

Lee, J, Hanley, J and Hopkins, V, *What Your Doctor Won't Tell You About Premenopause*, New York, Warners Books, 1999.

Lee Myeong, Soo, Huh, Hwa Jeong *et al.* 'Effects of emitted qi on in vitro natural killer,' *American Journal of Chinese Medicine*, 2001; 29: 17–22.

Leskowitz, E, 'Seasonal affective disorder and the yoga paradigm: a reconsideration of the role of the pineal gland,' *Medical Hypotheses*, 1990; 33: 155–158.

Liang, Shou-Yu, *Tachi-chuan: méthodes des 24 et 48 postures*, Noisy-sur-École, Budo Éditions, 2006.

Lipson, JG, 'We are the canaries: self-care in multiple chemical sensitivity sufferers,' Department of Community Health Systems, School of Nursing, University of California, San Francisco, *Qual Health Res, 2001; 11(1): 103–116.*

London Evening Standard, 'Orange to remove mobile mast from tower of doom,' www.thisislondon.co.uk/news/article-23407354-details/Orange+to+remove+mobile+mast+from+%27tower+of+doom%27%2C+where+cancer+rate+has+soared/article.do, accessed December 2011.

Lutz, A, Greischar, L, Rawling, N, Ricard, M and Davidson, R, 'Long-term meditators' self-induce high-amplitude gamma synchrony during mental practice,' *Proceedings of the National Academy of Sciences of the United States of America*, 2004; 101: 16369–16373.

McClelland, DC and Kirshnit, C, 'The effect of motivational arousal through films on salivary immunoglobulin A,' *Psychology and Health*, 1988; 2: 31–52.

McLelland, DC, Alexander, C and Marks, E, 'The need for power, stress, immune function, and illness among male prisoners,' *Journal of Abnormal Psychology*, 1983: 91: 61–70.

McColl, Mary Ann, *Spirituality and Occupational Therapy*, Ottawa, CAOT, 2003.

McGill University, 'The brain from top to bottom,' http://thebrain.mcgill.ca/, accessed December 2011.

McTaggart, L, *The Field*, New York, Harper Perennial, 2002.

Malpaux, B, Viguié, C, Thiéry, JC and Chemineau, P, 'Contrôle photopériodique de la reproduction,' *INRA Productions animales*, 1996; 9, 9–23.

Marchall, Katherine, 'Study: On sick leave,' *The Daily*, April 21, 2006; www.statcan.gc.ca/daily-quotidien/060421/dq060421d-eng.htm, accessed December 2011.

Maslach, C, 'Burn out: the cost of caring,' *Psychol Health*, 2001; 16(5): 607–111.

Massion, AO *et al.* 'Meditation, melatonin and breast/prostate cancer: hypothesis and preliminary data,' *Medical Hypotheses*, 1995; 4: 39–46.

Medline Plus, 'Vitamin A,' www.nlm.nih.gov/medlineplus/ency/article/002400.htm#References, accessed December 2011.

Mercola, J and Klindhardt, D, 'Mercury toxicity and systemic elimination agents,' *Journal of Nutritionnal and Environmental Medicine*, 2001; 11: 53–62.

Mertz, H, Morgan, V, Tanner, G, *et al.* 'Regional cerebral activation in irritable bowel syndrome,' *Gastroenterology*, 2000; 118: 842–848.

Modern Synopsis of Comprehensive Textbook of Psychiatry/III (3rd edition), Baltimore, Williams & Wilkins, 1981.

Mongeau, Serge, *La Simplicité volontaire, plus que jamais,* Montreal, Les Éditions Écosociété, 1998.

Montagu, A, *Touching: The Human Significance of the Skin* (2nd edition), New York, Harper & Row Publishers, 1978.

Musil, R, *The Confusions of Young Törless,* Pantheon Books, 1906.

Nadel, J and Decety, J, 'Résonance et agentivité,' *Cerveau & Psycho,* 2006; 13.

Office of Dietary Supplements, 'Vitamin and mineral supplement fact sheet,' *National Institute of Health,* http://ods.od.nih.gov/Health_Information/Vitamin_and_Mineral_Supplement_Fact_Sheets.aspx, accessed December 2011.

Ohya, T, Oikawa, N, Kawabata, R, Okabe, H and Kai S, ' Biophoton emission induced by osmotic stress in adzuki bean root,' *Jpn J Appl Phys Part 1,* 2003; 42(12): 7625–7628.

Or'ions, 'Bricard's Lawi, on www.info-systel.com/bricard_.en.html, accessed December 2011.

Padovan, Beatriz and Padovan-Catenne, Sônia 'Course notes,' Formation à la méthode Padovan de réorganisation neurofonctionnelle: Module II –Les fonctions orofaciales et leur rééducation, November 2005.

Pearsall, Paul, *Toxic Success: How to Stop Striving and Start Thriving,* Makawao, Inner Ocean Publishing, 2002.

Pearsall, Paul, *The Heart's Code,* New York, Broadway Books, 1998.

Pearsall, Paul, *Super Immunity,* Toronto, Ballantine Books, 1987.

Pelt, Jean-Maire and Séralini, Gilles-Éric, *Après nous le déluge,* Paris, Flammarion/Fayard, 2006.

Pert, Candace, *Molecules of Emotion,* New York, Touchstone, 1997.

Peverill, KI, Sparrow, LA and Reuter, DJ, 'Soil analysis: an interpretation manual,' Collingwood, Csiro Publishing, 1999.

Philpott, WH and Kalita, DK, *Brain Allergies* (2nd edition), Chicago, Keats Publishing, 2000.

Pitchford, Paul, *Healing with Whole Foods,* Berkeley, North Atlantic Books, 2002.

Popoviciu, L *et al.* 'Clinical, EEG, electromyographic and polysomnographic studies in restless legs syndrome caused by magnesium deficiency,' *Rom J Neurol Psychiatry,* 1993; 31: 55–61.

Porges, SW, 'Orienting in a defensive world: mammalian modification of our evolutionary heritage, a polyvagal theory,' *Psychophysiology,* 1995; 32: 301–318.

Provide, Robert, *Le Rire, sa vie, son œuvre,* Paris, Robert Laffont, 2003.

Radio Canada, 'Doit-on bannir les gras trans?,' *Maisonneuve en direct,* www.radio-canada.ca/radio/maisonneuve/19112004/42368.shtml, accessed December 2011.

Raloff, Janet, 'More waters test positive for drugs,' *Science News Online,* 2000; April 1, 17(0212).

Randolph, T and Moss, R, *An Alternative Approach to Allergies* (revised edition), New York, Harper and Row Publishers, 1990.

Ratey J, *A User's Guide to the Brain,* New York, First Vintage Books, 1994.

Rein, G and McCraty, R, 'Long-term effects of compassion on salivary IgA,' *Psychosomatic Medicine,* 1994; 56: 171–172.

Relyea, Rick A, 'Predator cues and pesticides: a double dose of danger for amphibians,' *Ecological Applications,* 2003; 13(6): 1515–1521.

RéuCARE, Réseau régional de prévention du risque cardio-vasculaire et rénale par l'éducation de patients dépistés, www.reucare.org, accessed December 2011.

Reuter-Lorenz, P and Davidson, Richard J, 'Deferential contributions of the two cerebral hemispheres to the perception of happy and sad faces,' *Neurophychologia*, 1981; 19(4): 609–613.

Ridha, Arem, *The Thyroid Solution,* Toronto, Random House Publishing, 1999.

Robinson, PE, Leczynski, BA, Kutz, FW, Remmers, JC, 'An evaluation of hexachlorobensene body-burden levels in the general population of the USA,' *IARC Sci Publ,* 1986; (77): 183–193.

Rona, Zoltan P, 'Altered immunity & leaky gut syndrome,' www.afpafitness.com/articles/altered-immunity-leaky-gut-syndrome/85/, accessed December 2011.

Rousseau, JJ, *Les Confessions de J.J. Rousseau,* Paris, Poiçot, 1797, livre IX.

Sagar, Stephen, *Restored Harmony: An Evidence Based Approach for Integrating Traditional Chinese Medicine into Complementary Cancer Care,* Etobicoke, Dreaming Dragon Fly Communications, 2001.

Sananés, R, *Homéopathie et langage du corps,* Paris, Laffont, 1982.

Schiff, BB and Rump, SA, 'Asymmetrical hemispheric activation and emotion: the effects of unilateral forced nostril breathing,' *Brain Cogn,* 1995; 29(3): 217–231.

Seligman, M, *Learned Optimism: How to Change Your Mind and Your Life,* New York, Vintage, 2006.

Selye, Hans, *The Stress of Life,* New York, McGraw-Hill Paperbacks, 1956.

Servan-Schreiber, David, *Healing without Freud or Prozac: Natural Approaches to Curing Stress, Anxiety and Depression without Drugs and without Psychoanalysis,* Emmaus, PA, Rodale Press, 2005.

Servan-Schreiber, David, *Guérir: le stress, l'anxiété et la dépression sans médicaments ni psychanalyse,* Paris, Laffont, 2003.

Siegel, BS, *Love, Medicine and Miracles,* New York, Harper & Row, 1986.

Shaw, CY and Tamura, GT, 'Air Ions And Human Comfort,' *Canadian Building Digests, NRC-IRC publications,* 1978: www.nrc-cnrc.gc.ca/eng/ibp/irc/cbd/building-digest-199.html, accessed December 2011.

Sheldrake, Rupert, *'Rupert Sheldrake, biologist and author,'* www.sheldrake.org/homepage.html, accessed December 2011.

Shulman, J, *Winning the Food Fight,* Etobicoke, John Wiley & Sons Canada, 2003.

Slawinski, J, Godlewski, M, Kwiecinska, T, Rajfur, Z, Sitko, D and Wierzuchowska, D, 'Stress-induced photon emission from perturbed organisms: biophoton emission, stress and disease,' *Experientia,* 1992; 48(11–12): 1041–1058.

Sperber, AD *et al.* 'Fibromyalgia in the irritable bowel syndrome: studies of prevalence and clinical implications,' *Am J Gastroenterol,* 1999; 94(12): 3541–3546.

Statistics Canada, *'Non-transmissible chronic diseases,'* www40.statcan.gc.ca/l01/ind01/l3_2966_1887-eng.htm?hili_none, accessed December 2011.

Stendhal, *De l'amour,* Fragments divers XLIII, Paris, Mongi l'Ainé, 1822.

Stetter, F and Kupper, S, 'Autogenic training: a meta-analysis of clinical outcome studies,' *Appl Psychophysiol Biofeedback,* 2002; 27(1): 45–98.

Stewart, John, *'Orthostatic hypotension: under diagnosed and under-treated?'* Conference paper, Montreal Neurological Institute, 2002.

Stoll, Andrew L, *The Omega-3 Connection,* New York, Simon & Schuster, 2001.

Taggart, HM *et al.* 'Effects of tai chi exercise on fibromyalgie symptoms and health-related quality of life,' *Orthop Nurs,* 2003; 22(5): 252–260.

Teitelbaum, Jacob, 'Online question and answer sessions,' *FM-CFS Canada,* www.fm-cfs.ca/QATeitelbaum. html, accessed December 2011.

The Times 'Where rivers run high on cocaine,' August 5, 2005.

Tollé, Eckhart, *The Power of Now,* Vancouver, Namaste Publishing Library, 2004.

Tollé, Eckhart, *Le pouvoir du moment présent,* Outremont, Ariane Éditions, 2000.

Tooley, GA *et al.* 'Acute increases in night-time plasma melatonin levels following a period of meditation,' *Biological Psychology,* 2000; 53: 69–78.

Totheoh, Gailon, 'What's in that? How food affects behaviour,' *CBC News Science & Medical,* July 1, 2008; www.cbn.com/CBNnews/353246.aspx, accessed December 2011.

Townsend, E, Banks, S, Multari, L and Naugh, A, *OT Guidelines for Client-Centred Practice,* Toronto, CAOT, 1991.

Trombly, CA, *Occupational Therapy for Physical Dysfunction* (2nd edition), Baltimore, Williams & Wilkins, 1983.

Trudel, Louis and Saint-Jean, Micheline, 'Réadaptation au travail après un diagnostic d'épuisement professionnel: rôle émergent de l'ergothérapeute,' CAOT preconference workshop, May 30, 2006.

Tuttle, Dave, 'Keeping a dangerous hormone in check,' *Life Extension,* July 2004.

Vollaard, EJ and Clasener, HA, 'Colonization resistance,' *Antimicrobial Agents and Chemotherapy,* 1994; 38, 409–414.

Vulgaris Médical, 'Acide pantothenique,' www.vulgaris-medical.com/front/?p=index_fiche&id_article=139, accessed December 2011.

Vulgaris Médical, 'Vitamine B2,' www.vulgaris-medical.com/front/?p=index_fiche&id_article=4817, accessed December 2011.

Wass, J and Shalet, S, *Oxford Textbook of Endocrinology and Diabetes,* Bath, Oxford University Press, 2002.

Wayne, PM *et al.* 'Can tai chi improve vestibulopathic postural control?,' *Arch Phy Med Rehab,* 2004; 85.

Whorwell, PJ *et al.* 'Physiological effects of emotion: assessment via hypnosis,' *Lancet,* 1992; 340(8811): 69–72.

Wilson, EK, 'Fields of genes,' *Chem Eng News,* 24 March 2003: 27–29.

Wilson, James L. *Adrenal Fatigue: The 21st Century Stress Syndrome,* Petaluma, CA, Smart Publications, 2001.

Wing, L, 'The definition and prevalence of autism: a review,' *European Journal of Child & Adolescent Psychiatry,* 1993; 2(2): 61–74.

World Research Foundation, 'The electrical pattern of life; the work of Harold S. Burr,' www.wrf.org/men-women-medicine/dr-harold-s-burr.php, accessed December 2011.

Xu, D, Hong, Y, Li, J and Chan, K, 'Effect of taichi exercises on proprioception of ankle and knee joints in old people,' Department of Sport, Science and Physical Education, and Department of Orthopedics and Traumatology, The Chinese University of Hong Kong, Feb. 2003.

Zervas, Eleftherios *et al.* 'Reduced intracellular Mg concentration in patients with acute asthma,' *Chest,* 2003; 123: 113–118.

Zinker, J, *Se créer par la Gestalt,* Montreal, Éditions de l'Homme, 1981.

Further Reading

Barr Murray, L and Kiernan, John A, *The Human Nervous System* (4th edition), Philadelphia, Harper and Row, 1983.

Berk, L *et al.* 'Immune system changes during humor associated laughter,' *Clinical Research*, 1989; 39: 124A.

Bunzel, B *et al.* 'Does Changing the heart mean changing personality? a retrospective inquiry on 47 heart transplant patients,' *Quality of Life Research*, 1992; 1: 251–256.

Canatarogly, A *et al.* 'Prevalence of fibromyalgia in patients with irritable bowel syndrome,' *Am J Gastroenterology*, 1999; 94(12): 3541–3546.

Chalko, TJ, 'Is chance of choice the essence of nature,' *NU Journal of Discovery*, March 2001; vol. 2.

Cho, ZH, Chung, SC, Jones, JP *et al.* 'New findings of the correlation between acupoints and corresponding brain cortices using functional MRI,' *Proc Natl Acad Sci USA*, 1998; 95: 2670–2673.

Christiansen, C, 'Defining lives: occupation as identity: an essay on competence, coherence, and the creation of meaning,' Eleanor Clarke Slagle Lecture, *American Journal of Occupational Therapy*, 1999; 53: 547–558.

Coico, Richard, Sunshine, Geoffrey, Benjamini, Eli, *Immunology: A Short Course*, New York, John Wiley and Sons, 2003.

Cynkin, Simme, *Occupational Therapy: Toward Health through Activities*, Boston, Little, Brown and Company, 1979.

Diamond, John, *Life Energy*, St Paul, Paragone House, 1990.

Doidge, Norman, *The Brain that Changes Itself,* New York, Viking, 2007.

Dunton, WR, *Reconstruction Therapy*, Philadelphia, WB, 1919.

Dyer, Wayne, *The Power of Intention,* Carlsbad, Hay House, 2004.

English, Thomas, 'A piece of my mind: skeptical of sceptics,' *JAMA*, 1991; 265: 964.

Feldenkrais, Moshe, *Awareness through Movement: Health Exercises for Personal Growth*, New York, HarperCollins, 1990.

Ferland, Francine, *Pour parent débordés et en manque d'énergie*, Montreal, Éditions CHU Ste-Justine, 2006.

Fletcher, W, *Beating the 24/7, How Business Leaders Achieve a Successful WorkLife Balance*, Etobicoke, John Wiley & Sons Canada, 2002.

Gawain, Shakti, *Creative Visualization Meditations* (2nd edition), Novato, New World Library, 2002.

Hagerty, John J Jr *et al.* 'Prevalence of antithyroid antibodies in mood disorders,' *Depression and Anxiety*, 1997; 5(2): 91–96.

Hanley, Jesse Lynn, *Tired of Being Tired,* New York, Berkley, 2001.

Henley, WN and Koehnle, TJ, 'Thyroid hormone, neural tissue and mood modulation,' *World J Biol Psychiatry*, 2001; 2(2): 59–69.

Jurczynska, J and Zieleniewski, W, 'Clinical implications of occurrence of antithyroid antibodies in pregnant women and in the postpartum period.' *Przegl Lek*, 2004; 61(8): 864–867.

Kaplan, H and Sadock, B, *Modern Synopsis of Comprehensive Textbook of Psychiatry/III* (3rd edition), Baltimore, Williams & Wilkins, 1981.

Kermode-Scott, Barbara, 'To be a healer: Dr. Ruth Wilson treads a path to primary care reform,' *Le médecin de famille canadien, Mississauga, CMFC*, August 2001: 1683.

Law, Mary, 'Autism spectrum disorders and occupational therapy,' Briefing to the Senate Standing Committee on Social Affairs, Science and Technology, *CAOT*, Nov. 2006.

Mason, GA, Walker, CH and Prange, AJ Jr, 'L-triiodothyronine: is this peripheral hormone a central neurotransmitter,' *Neuropsychopharmacology*, 1993; 8(3): 253–258.

Nemeroff, CB, Simon, JS, Haggerty, JJ Jr and Evans, DL, 'Antithyroid antibodies in depressed patients,' *Am J Psychiatry*, 1985; 142: 840–843.

Newmark, ST *et al.* 'Adrenocortical response to marathon running,' *Journal of Clinical Endocrinology & Metabolism*, 1976; 42: 393–394.

Panossian, AG, 'Adaptogens: a historical overview and perspective,' *Natural Pharmacy*, 2003; 7(4): 1, 19–20.

Reichenberg, A. *et al.* 'Advancing paternal age and autism,' *Arch Gen Psychiatry*, 2006; 63: 1026–1032.

Riverdale, Sher L, 'Role of thyroid hormones in the effects of selenium on mood, behaviour, and cognitive function,' *Med Hypotheses*, 2001; 57(4): 480–483.

Rotton, J and Shatts, M, 'Effects of state humour expectancies, and choice on postsurgical mood and self-medication: a field experiment,' *Journal of Applied Social Psychology*, 1996; 26, 1775–1794.

Townsend, E, Banks, S, Multari, L and Naugh, A, *OT Guidelines For Client-Centred Practice*, Toronto, CAOT, 1991.

Scheibner, Viera, 'Effects of adjuvants in vaccinations,' *Nexus*, Dec. 2000; 8(1) and Feb. 2001; 8(2).

Selye, Hans, *Stress without Distress*, New York, J B Lippincott, 1974.

Schumacher, EF, *Small Is Beautiful*, Contretemps/Le Seuil, Paris, 1978.

Thie, John and Thie, Matthew, *Touch for Health: A Practical Guide to Natural Health with Acupressure Touch*, Camarillo, De Vorss Publications, 2005.

Tikhoniv, VP *et al.* 'Complex therapeutical effect of ionized air: stimulation of the immune system and decrease in excessive serotonin. H/sub2/as a link between the two counterparts,' *Plasma Science IEEE*, August 2004; 32(4), Part 2: 1661–1667.

Vander, A, Sherman, J and Luciano, D, *Human Physiology: The Mechanisms of Body Function* (3rd edition), New York, McGraw-Hill Book Company, 1980.

Vaughan, GM *et al.* 'Nocturnal elevation of plasma melatonin and urinary 5- hydroxyindoleacetic acid in young men: attempts at modification by brief changes in environmental lighting and sleep and by autonomic drugs,' *J Clinical Endocrinology Metabolism*, 1976; 42: 752–764.

Vimy, MJ, Luft, AJ and Lorscheider, FL, 'Estimation of mercury body burden from dental amalgam computer simulation of a metabolic compartment model,' *J Dent Res*, 1986; 65(12): 1415–1419.

Wakefield, Jerome *et al.* 'Extending the bereavement exclusion for major depression to other losses,' *Arch Gen Psychiatry*, 2007; 64: 433–440.

Index